KATY

A Fight for Life

By the same author

PAST IMPERFECT

THE JOAN COLLINS BEAUTY BOOK

KATY

A Fight for Life

Joan Collins

LONDON
VICTOR GOLLANCZ LTD
1982

British Library Cataloguing in Publication Data

Collins, Joan
  Katy.
  1. Children – Wounds and injuries – Personal narratives
  2. Critically ill – Personal narratives
  I. Title
  362.1'971028   RD93.5C4
  ISBN 0-575-03111-5

Photoset in Great Britain by
Rowland Phototypesetting Limited, Bury St Edmunds, Suffolk
and printed by St Edmundsbury Press, Bury St Edmunds, Suffolk

This book is for Katy, and for all the other Katys and their parents who find themselves in this unfortunate situation. I hope these words will help them, and that they will not give up the fight—as Katy did not.

Acknowledgements

Many, many people helped Ron and me during our ordeal—friends, doctors, nurses and other hospital staff. On advice from my publishers, I have had to omit many of their names, but they know who they are and that they have Ron's and my eternal gratitude.

We are grateful to the Souvenir Press Ltd for permission to include an extract from *Living After a Stroke* by Diana Law and Barbara Paterson (published in the Human Horizon Series).

J.C.

List of Illustrations

Eleven weeks: Katy visits hospital.

Joan and Katy present some equipment to the Premature Baby Unit.

She's getting better all the time!

The caravan Joan and Ron lived in for six weeks.

Following page 128

Christmas 1980.

Five months: "Our beautiful Katy is beginning to emerge again."

Six months: She starts to show her old vigorous personality.

She runs properly for the first time.

Back at school.

Ten months: Happy Ninth Birthday!

Eleven months: Katy's school sports day.

One year.

The day Katy passed a school entrance examination.

Thirteen months: With Sacha.

Fourteen months.

Fifteen months: "She has come a long, long way."

Any photographs not individually credited in the plate sections come from Joan Collins' private photograph albums.

Foreword

Serious life-threatening injury to a child is one of the most distressing events parents may have to face. To the grief and distress of illness is added anger at the event having taken place, and guilt at not having been able to prevent it. What all parents seek is reassurance that their child will recover, and to know what they, who know the child best, can do to help. Doctors caring for a child with serious injuries are therefore faced with a dilemma. They may not, in all honesty, be able to give what the parents so desperately need—a confident prediction of survival and recovery—without evoking further anger and guilt if events prove them wrong. Clearly hope must always be given but the nuances of guarded predictions are often misunderstood or forgotten during the early days so full of distress. It is significant that Joan's diary only starts on Day 14, when Katy's survival seemed certain, and there is no real account of the numerous conversations with doctors before that.

Sadly, even today medicine has little to offer in treatment of brain injury, and the outcome is largely determined by the severity of the initial injury. All modern methods, including life-support systems, provide little more than supportive maintenance of the body until the brain recovers, and not all outcomes are as happy as the one described here. During this period most parents can, and should, be involved as much as possible, and after

11

the first few days can make a major contribution with care and stimulation as Katy's parents did. Joan drew much of her hope from the letters of the Davison family, who had recently gone through a similar experience. Hopefully this book will do the same for other parents.

R. D. Illingworth, FRCS
Central Middlesex Hospital
January 1982

Prologue

I hadn't really wanted to go to Paris. It was August 1980, and I was feeling slightly put out about having to drag myself across the Channel—even to meet the fabled designer M. Romaine de Tertoff Erté. He wasn't able to come and see me because he was too busy. Well, I was busy too, and although I was greatly excited by the prospect of M. Erté designing my four costumes for the forthcoming production of *The Last of Mrs Cheyney*, I was exhausted from two years of almost non-stop work.

Tara, my sixteen-year-old daughter from my previous marriage, had recently arrived from Los Angeles. Sacha, my fourteen-year-old son, and Robert, my husband Ron's seventeen-year-old son, were both staying in our tiny house in Mayfair for the summer holidays, so it was a full house. I was truly happy to have all my children with me.

It had been a busy two years: two movies in a row followed by rehearsing and performing *The Last of Mrs Cheyney* in Chichester for six months, commuting by train and car. Then I had gone straight from the closing night at Chichester into rehearsals and shooting for *Tales of the Unexpected*, which was basically a two-hander with a tough shooting schedule during the unusually hot summer. Rehearsals for the West End production of *The Last of Mrs Cheyney* were due to start in the first week of September 1980 so we were excitedly preparing for our August holiday at our home in California.

But first I had to go to Paris.

Tara had never seen Paris, and Ron and I decided it would

be fun to show her the sights. Fiona Aitken (Katy's nanny) and Robert and Sacha were to travel to Los Angeles on 2nd August. Katy—Ron's and my only child from our marriage— would stay for two days with her best schoolfriend, Georgina.

When I called Georgina's mother to ask her if Katy could stay for the weekend (as I had many times before), I was slightly worried when she said that she was driving to Ascot to visit her sister, but would love Katy to come. I felt a twinge of apprehension as I asked her if she would please drive care- fully, and she assured me, laughingly, that she was a very careful driver. Katy was very precious to us, as were all our children. Katy was angry that she couldn't fly with the boys and Fiona to Los Angeles, but I had this absolute phobia about her travelling on an airplane without either Ron or me accom- panying her, and it was totally impossible to take her to Paris for just forty-eight hours.

By the time we dropped her off at Georgina's home in the morning she was her usual happy, laughing self again, and with many blown kisses and assurances that we would come back soon—"with a big box of chocolates from Paris"—she, and we, felt at ease.

At two o'clock in the morning on 2nd August 1980, in a lushly appointed suite in the Hotel Lancaster, the telephone rang. I was asleep, and so was Tara in the connecting room. Ron had gone to a movie and had just returned. I sleepily heard him answer the phone. I heard him say, "An accident— Katy? How bad?"

I struggled out of sleep and he looked at me with a stunned expression on his face.

"It's Katy—she's been hit by a car. She's . . . critical—a head injury."

"No!" I heard myself scream. "No, no, no!" I wanted to go back to sleep and wake up again. This was a nightmare. It *must* be a nightmare. "Not my baby, not Katy!" I started to scream and thrash about. All my reason went. I was just like an animal. I had no control—just unbearable agony and the frustration of being away from our beloved little girl at such a time.

Tara came rushing in, dreadfully frightened at the sight of her mother almost out of control, and tried to comfort me. I felt physically sick, and was. All the time I begged them to wake me up from this dream. Ron started to call the airlines to try and get us out of Paris. I opened the fridge and found four or five assorted miniature bottles of brandy and scotch. I drank two or three and calmed down. We had to be practical and keep our heads. We had to get out of Paris. We had to push thoughts of what had happened to Katy out of our minds and concentrate on finding a way of getting to her. Fast!

We called the hospital and spoke to a doctor. He had a foreign accent and didn't sound too optimistic. He put Katy's headmistress on the phone. When the hospital or police hadn't been able to find any of our immediate family (Jackie, my sister, was in Los Angeles; my brother and my father out to dinner), they called John Gold (a close friend whose children also went to Katy's school) and he had called the headmistress. She had rushed over and had been with Katy ever since, holding her hand and giving support.

She was comforting. Over the long-distance wires her soothing voice seemed to allay our fears temporarily. She acted as if Katy was in safe hands and would be okay.

We called the British and American Embassies in Paris trying to find a way to get out. They could do nothing. Neither could the concierge. Neither could BEA or Air France. We were stuck in Paris for at least another seven hours until a nine a.m. flight to London.

In those hours anything could happen to Katy. It was unthinkable.

Icy calm descended on us. We called several friends with

15

private planes. They were all away. Of course. It was 2nd August. Everyone was on holiday. I called my father in London.

"I don't suppose Roger Whittaker could come and get us?" I begged helplessly, knowing that Roger had a pilot's licence.

Daddy was dubious. It was Saturday night/Sunday morning and if Roger had been out and had had even one drink he couldn't pilot the plane. But Daddy said he would try to reach him.

Half a nail-biting hour went by. I lay on the sofa numb with shock and apprehension. Tara put ice all over me and tried to comfort me. Ron paced up and down being very strong, but he too was biting his nails.

At 3.30 in the morning a wonderfully calm voice called.

"Joan, it's Roger. Be at Le Bourget at 5.30—I'm coming to get you!"

In the next two hours every kind of emotion raced through our minds. Elation that we were finally getting out of Paris, despair and frustration that we were not with our daughter at this critical time.

Guilt. How could we have gone off to Paris and left her— even with people we trusted?

Fury. *How* did it happen? and *why*? What carelessness allowed it? Whose fault was it?

Grief. Our baby lying in hospital in what condition we couldn't imagine. And finally the dreadful, awful, nagging fear that we would be too late. That she would be dead by the time we arrived at the hospital.

For two hours we paced the suite. Tara, Ron and I comforted each other but I was by far in the worst shape. I felt numb with shock and kept giving myself ridiculous things to do—as when you are a child you jump across the pavement and mustn't tread on any cracks, and if you did not something good would happen. So I felt that if I threw up—was sick—

Katy would live. It sounds ridiculous but a voice in my head, the old ingrained actor's voice of superstition, kept telling me to do this.

As we raced through the darkened streets of Paris in a limousine conjured up by the hotel concierge, the same voice kept telling me again, "If you make the green traffic light before it turns to red, she'll live. . . ."

"No, no." I squeezed my eyes shut. I didn't want to have contests with this superstitious inner voice. I held on to Ron who was like a rock. Very strong, very calm. Inside, though, I could see he was in agony. Katy was his only daughter. He worshipped her.

We arrived at Le Bourget at five. It was still dark. The ground staff knew nothing about Roger's arrival. Ron did his strong act while Tara and I walked round and round the tiny airport lounge. I smoked constantly, and wept. I was in pretty awful shape. I still wore a ridiculously inappropriate dress I'd bought in Paris the day before. Red and white, candy striped like a tent, white sandals and a sun visor. It was what I had put out to travel in. It seemed so wrong but it didn't matter.

We searched the sky for hours it seemed. No plane. The sky started to lighten. Dawn was coming. Was my baby still alive?

We called the hospital. My brother, Bill, was there with Robin Guild, another friend. They assured us she was holding her own, but I know they were trying to make us feel better. The more snippets of information that were revealed, the worse it seemed.

Brain Injury. The meaning of that was not clear.

Coma. Was it just a long sleep or was it, as I had heard, the closest thing to death?

I closed my mind. I did not know what to expect. I refused to think the unthinkable.

Tara and I paced around the tarmac for what seemed an eternity, gazing at the ever-lightening sky. She was brave, my

17

sixteen-year-old girl. It must have been hell for her to think of what was happening with the clarity of adolescence.

"Don't worry, Mummy," she kept reassuring me. "Katy's a big strong kid—nothing's going to get her—you must believe that, Mummy, you must."

She gave me support as we waited the endless wait.

When Ron and I looked into each other's eyes all we saw was stark terror. We could not speak too much. We held each other. We cried. Occasionally I would rush to the loo to be sick again. I have only been sick about three times in my life. It was odd. I smoked a thousand cigarettes and prayed.

Roger Whittaker's plane finally landed. By this time Ron's nails were bitten to the knuckle, and I felt close to a complete nervous breakdown. I fell on to Roger's chest and burst into tears, although I felt there could not be too many tears left to shed. He shook me like a Dutch uncle and told me to shape up. Not to imagine the unthinkable, to think positive. He almost shouted at me and strangely it calmed me down.

We hardly spoke during the hour-and-a-half journey in the tiny plane back to London Airport. Ron and I held hands. He was trying hard not to give in to his terror. He was trying to be strong for me. For Katy. If there still was a Katy.

We drank some coffee from a Thermos flask Roger had brought. I tried to blot out my thoughts and started to pray to God. To a God I had never really acknowledged existed. Not that I believed he didn't—I was agnostic. Now I prayed for my daughter's life with all my might.

At London Airport they hastened us through Customs. Bill and Robin were waiting. Tara and I went with Bill, and Robin insisted on taking Ron in his car.

We sped through the deserted summer Sunday streets. Bill prepared me for the fact that they had cut off all Katy's hair. He kept assuring me she was going to be all right. I felt he was keeping the real truth from me by telling me this detail. We passed a graveyard. Thousands and thousands of grey and white stones. I shuddered and turned away. Tara was very quiet and I tried to comfort her. We held each other's hands tightly. She was eight years older than Katy but Katy adored her big sister and I know Tara loved her too.

We tore through the hospital and came to the Intensive Care Unit. I don't know what I thought I was going to see, but I didn't believe what I saw. My baby was lying in a brightly-lit room naked to the waist. Her long blonde hair was gone. It was hacked off to the skull. She was white. Bluish white. She was tiny. Instead of a husky eight-year-old, she looked like a tiny infant. She had tubes in her nose, in her wrists; from under her bed-sheet she had a ventilator life-support system down her throat to help her breathing. She was still as stone, her eyes closed, her breathing a whisper. Her left hand was clenched and bent above her head. I took her right hand in mine and squeezed it.

"Katy, darling, Mummy's here. I'm here, darling. If you can hear me squeeze my hand. Please Katy, squeeze my hand." From the depths of her being, from the part of her brain that was working, she squeezed my hand. I knew she had heard. I knew she would survive.

To be what, though, we did not know. Ron came in a few minutes after me. He too spent some time at Katy's bedside. While he was with her I saw Dr Lionel Balfour-Lynn, Katy's paediatrician, who had been present at her birth.

"What are her chances?" I asked.

Tears filled his eyes. "Of survival, sixty–forty—against."

I burst into tears of disbelief. Ron came out of the Intensive Care Unit and took me to the back door. We held each other tightly and sobbed together. We made a vow to each other. She *could not* die. She *would not*. We would do everything possible to make her live. We would not accept what the prognosis was, however pessimistic. We would pour into her our love, our faith, our prayers, our strength, our optimism, our utter positivity. All this we talked about in sobbing whispers at the back door of the ICU, surrounded by shelves full of shrouds.

Five minutes later we went in to see our daughter again. I had dried my tears and Ron had dried his. She would not see us cry again. From now on what Katy would receive from us was total positive input and the *firm belief* that she was going to live and that she was going to recover.

The first day had begun.

After two weeks I began to write a diary, partly to relieve the unbearable tension and partly to record Katy's day-by-day progress. The idea of publishing it never entered my head. But now I have decided that it *should* be published, because I know it can help other people in the way that the letters from other parents who had been through similar nightmares helped Ron and me.

Joan Collins
Los Angeles
December 1981

Now that the full horror of the past two weeks of Katy's accident has passed and I feel confidence and strength that she is going to pull through completely, I feel I can put down some words about her day-by-day progress.

DAY 1: *3rd August 1980:* 2 a.m.

In Paris we heard the ghastly nightmare news that our beloved child had been hit by a car and was in a critical condition in the Intensive Care Unit at the Central Middlesex Hospital, Acton. We had only left her for one night and the horror of being trapped in Paris, knowing she had had the accident over six hours ago and being powerless to go to her will never leave me. I screamed when I heard Ron talking on the phone, and woke my daughter Tara who came running in. There were no scheduled flights from Paris at this time of night, but at last a miracle arrived in the shape of Roger Whittaker, who flew his own plane from Stansted to Le Bourget at six a.m. to pick us up. My thoughts from this time until I saw my baby are indescribable. I tried to keep my mind a blank, couldn't consider what the possibilities were—dead—maimed—a vegetable. I screamed silently and not so silently to myself in the agonizing time (six hours) until I stood at her bedside. I can't believe it. I just *can't*. She looked so tiny in the big hospital bed, and there were tubes and support systems everywhere. Her long blonde hair had all gone, her eyes were closed, machines breathed for her and fed her. I squeezed her little hand and told her, "Mama's here," and I felt a faint squeeze back. I'm sure she heard me and responded. I talked

21

to her for about ten minutes, as much as I could without breaking down. I don't know what I said.

Dr Lionel Balfour-Lynn was outside with my brother Bill and our friend, the designer Robin Guild. He told me her chances of survival were sixty–forty against and they hadn't expected her to survive the night. I broke down completely. How could this happen to Katy? Strong, beautiful, clever, funny kid, compassionate, wilful—our divine child. What horrendous twist of fate gave her this?

Ron and I tried to pull ourselves together. We had to do something to help our baby, but we didn't know what and no one at the hospital gave us any advice on what strategy to take. Katy's initial response to my squeezing her hand was a positive sign, Ron and I decided, even though the nurses were sceptical and thought it was a reflex action. Even if there is only a tiny ray of hope we have decided to talk to Katy *all* the time and try and keep active that part of her brain which is still working. It would reassure her that we were there, that we loved her. In some way I believed that our voices were reaching her, helping her, but I was confused and hysterical away from her.

Ron wept too but he became strong when we sat by little Katy. We must be strong for her. She needs us now more than ever.

DAY 2

I spent all night at Katy's side talking to her, and today there is a blur of hope and agony. Mr Illingworth, her neurosurgeon, sees a flicker of improvement. They won't tell us much about the ultimate outcome, though. All we want now is for her to survive.

The press have been driving us mad, calling constantly, and photographers lurk in the corridor snapping me with long-distance lenses. The hospital have had to bring in guards. Our PR has to cope. He said one tabloid actually wanted a photo of me at the bottom of Katy's bed in the Intensive Care Unit— how sick can you get? The papers play up the story rather a lot. I can understand them doing it, but at the same time I resent it.

DAY 3

Our optimism builds a tiny bit. Each hour means more hope. The Intensive Care Unit team are magnificent. Many friends come to visit. Letters, cards and telegrams pour in. All are full of compassion, love, and above all tremendous *hope*. I realize how many people love Katy. And why not indeed?—she is entirely special. We talk to her *constantly*. Some of the letters are from men and women who have been in similar situations. They tell me what to expect. They give me hope. All say the same things: *love*, faith, and a constant input of energy and stimulation.

Dear Joan and Ron,

I just had to write and let you know that you are in our thoughts at this terrible time in your lives and my heart really aches for you because you see Joan I was in the same position myself just as little time ago as three and a half months. I know the horror of sitting hour after hour at your little girl's bedside. For the first three days I did not wash, have anything to eat or change my clothes, it's like a dream but you don't wake up.

So Joan my dear you are going to have to be strong the strongest you've ever been in your life but it's hard sitting telling story after story trying to remember anything stimu-lating to talk about for hours on end.

They told us they did not know of what outcome there was for our Tracy but after she came out of the ICU and on to the ward at least she was alive and that was all we wanted at first. And Joan like any parent once we knew she was going to live we wanted more. So we went to work on her like we had not done in our lives before because where there's life there's hope.

We stayed at the hospital for three months. She was in the ICU for six days, slowly so slowly we did not dare to hope for more she came back to us just like your Katy will to you. Our Tracy was unconscious for nearly six weeks. Alan (my husband) and I put a lot of work into her and the results are so slow when you leave the bedside you have a good cry but never beside little Katy's bed because I'm convinced that they know what is going on but the body has not got the strength to face life till it's ready to.

Our Tracy is going back to school after the six weeks. Her speech is a little slow but that will come with time. We had to learn her to talk and toilet train, feed her and walk, we were told to expect a long long job and then they just could not tell us anything they just said waiting is the thing. Well Joan, as I say it's only three and a half months ago and I wish you could see her—every morning she's up first playing records and keeping everyone awake, she's got so much life in her, she's running around just like she was before.

When she comes in I'm going to ask her to drop you a line, her writing is still a little shaky but that will come with time as well.

Joan our Tracy had her hair shaved off as I think your little Katy will have but it's growing now and I have took the liberty of sending two photos one taken just before the accident and one just a fortnight ago, keeping hold of a friend's baby who she called Tracy after our Tracy.

Joan I know you don't feel like writing letters but if you would like me to keep in touch as we had to go by scratch and I'm sure we would be able to support you a little being in the same boat ourselves. I've put a self addressed envelope inside as I know you'll not want to be bothered with stamps and things.

And I hope you don't mind me writing but I thought I

would tell you about our Tracy as I'm sure you already know love can overcome anything and I'm sure it won't be very long before those thin little arms that are lying limp now will be flung round your neck again in the very near future.

I have not gone into great detail about our Tracy I just wanted to let you know that you do get results but it's a slow job and our Tracy is living proof of that. So if you would like to know how we went about it I would be very pleased to go along with you with the different stages Katy will go through.

So I hope I've helped a little as I also am sitting by Katy's bedside with you in thought. It's a very true saying you only know what it's like if you've gone through it yourself.

Mr and Mrs Davison

PS I'm not very good at spelling I hope you understand it all right.

DAY 4

We feel more confident now she will survive. Her hands move and she is over the first forty-eight hours—the most crucial time. I talk to Alana Stewart in Los Angeles who tells me about a psychic who has been praying for Katy. I call her. She is absolutely *positive* Katy will pull through and even though she may have some sort of disability she will overcome it with therapy. She says she sees a shining light around Katy, like a halo. She says to get a minister from the Pentecostal Church to anoint her and say a special prayer for her. She says she sees a break in the crisis in fifty-eight hours.

Ron has to give a press conference, then they have promised to leave us alone. I can't. I'm still too close to tears all the time. Only when I'm with Katy am I completely in control of myself and full of laughter and happiness to transmit to her. Ron does an excellent job of talking to dozens of people, although it is a tremendous effort for him. He has not slept for more than an hour or two for the past five days. I'm worried about him. He is such a strong man physically and emotionally, and he is giving me so much support in this—what many people seem to think is a futile exercise. I will *not* stop talking to Katy, and stimulating her little hands, face and feet by touch. Something tells me it is the right thing to do and it is going to work. My voice is becoming hoarse. Whenever I leave her side I rush to the little room the hospital has set aside for relatives of those in intensive care and I smoke three or four cigarettes, one after the other, and drink several cups of coffee or some wine from a bottle. I feel slightly demented.

DAY 6 or 7

Mr Illingworth decides she has progressed enough to remove the tube down her throat which is attached to the ventilating machine which aids her breathing. This is a very daring move as it means that if she can't breathe—or if she inhales vomit— or—I can't bear to think of it. . . . The other doctors didn't think that she was ready to breathe on her own, that her brain wouldn't give the right signals to her system, so there was an emergency team on hand ready to perform a tracheotomy. But when the tube was removed we heard raspy sounds coming from Katy's throat—she was breathing! It was fantastic! It is a *positive* step and means a tiny bit of progress, and for the first time Ron and I heave the faintest sigh of relief. She has an enormous sort of boil on her lip from the rubbing of the tube but this gets better in twelve hours—a sign that she has good recuperative powers. Ron warns me, however, that if Katy should suddenly develop breathing difficulties, not having the ventilator connected could present imminent disaster. I refuse to contemplate this. By now I refuse to contemplate the possibility of Katy's death. There is a vast graveyard that we pass on the way into central London. Whenever we pass it I close my eyes and pretend it doesn't exist.

Ron and I are sleeping and living at the hospital in a tiny cramped room. I am the object of great interest—the famous sex symbol who looks like a hundred miles of unpaved road. I don't bother about my appearance, never even have time to clean my teeth. But I don't give a damn who sees me. I only care about pouring all my energy and strength into Katy.

I think perhaps being an actress is, in some macabre way, being a slight help to me in this ghastly nightmare. I actually sometimes psych myself into believing it's not really happening—*you're playing a role, Joan, this is someone else's life you're portraying*—I know it sounds daft but my strength is what Katy needs and I will give it to her, come what may.

I go to the chapel and pray. I get the minister from the Pentecostal Church to come and give her the blessing the American psychic wanted. Also the hospital chaplain says a prayer for her, Ron's mother has a service for her in Los Angeles, Johnny Gold's mother has asked the rabbi to do a service, and Jan's mother—a Portuguese Catholic—has had a special Mass said. Everyone is praying for her complete recovery. The energy is strong. I feel a positivity but I can't bear to go home. I can't bear to look at the photographs of my gorgeous, laughing, blonde-haired little girl. I love *this* little girl with the punk-rock haircut and the tubes in her. The other Katyana has gone away for a little while. She will return, I know.

DAY 7

The hospital wants the room where we have been living for the past six days, as there are others who need it. Ron called Guido Cohen, who runs Twickenham Studios, and he told us to contact Willie Fonfe, the head of Willie's Wheels, to hire a trailer to live in while we keep our vigil. Willie said he would send his men to hook up the best caravan he had available, and would loan it to us for as long as we needed it. He was disappointed that all his luxury caravans were out on hire for the film *Reds* and he had only a modest one. For us it is a godsend. The hospital suggested we hook into their water and power systems to save the noise of a generator, and the phone company were wonderful in installing a much-needed telephone immediately. We have a fridge and a stove, a bathroom with a shower and a chemical toilet, and a living area containing a double bed. A kind chap from Radio Rentals sent us a television to help make the moments away from Katy's bed less painful. I have seen *Dallas*—for the first time ever.

All Katy's old nannies come to visit, a tribute to what a wonderful kid she is. There are cards and letters from so many people.

DAY 8

As I came back from buying the Sunday papers Ron appeared excitedly and yelled at me from the caravan, "She's opened her eyes!" I rushed over and her eyes were indeed open. There's no expression in them and she's still in a coma, but it is *great* progress. Even Mr Illingworth smiled! This occurred exactly sixty hours after I spoke to the psychic in Los Angeles who saw a break in the crisis in fifty-eight hours.

Later: We have had a terrible fright. Katy stopped breathing today. Apparently she had a muscular spasm which seized up her respiratory system. The sister in charge started her breathing again within seconds, and because she was still attached to the life-support machines, which gave the alarm, the resuscitation team was alerted immediately. There was no real danger but it was a horrifying episode. When she is moved to the Children's Ward she won't be attached to all the machines.

28

She is more helpless than a new-born baby now—she can't even cry and has no way of showing she is uncomfortable or distressed. This evening Ron and I decided we must watch her constantly. We decided that he will be with her at night and I will do the day-shift. He says I am better at talking to her and we think she should have lots more stimulation during her "waking" hours.

DAY 9

They are going to give Katy a brain scan and then move her from Intensive Care to the Children's Ward. I am nervous as hell about the scan—all that radiation*—but Ron goes with her as I have to give my one and only interview—to a sympathetic Shaun Usher from the *Daily Mail*. The press have laid siege to the hospital and this may relieve it a little. I also want to show my appreciation and admiration for the hospital staff, and also to try to help other parents, if I can, as so many have helped me with their letters. I know we are not alone. It seems unbelievable, the amount of children this happens to each year—some figures are as high as seven or eight thousand.

One of the male nurses, Joe, made a great sacrifice. Because Katy moved her head when they were trying to scan it, he held it for three doses of radiation. My faith in the goodness of my fellow man is becoming stronger all the time. Every day brings a letter of hope and comfort from another parent. I contacted Mrs Davison and we spoke to her little Tracy, who sounds fine if a little slow in speech, but her accident was only three and a half months ago.

The doctors still cannot predict an end to this—they said initially that the coma could be at least six weeks. But this Katy

* Mr Illingworth has since pointed out that the radiation dose from the scan is very low and the risk is minimal, particularly compared to the invaluable information the scan provides.

of ours is a fighter and her eyes remain open more every day although the expression is still blank. It's like having a new-born baby and being thrilled with its every new movement. Ron says she is re-born and starting from scratch again.

She is moved to the Children's Ward, which is cheerful and full of jolly little leg injuries, premature babies and sweet nurses. A show of visitors arrive. Jade Jagger and Jerry Hall bring a gorgeous talking doll and Doug Hayward and Lucy Mills a bottle of scotch—*that* I really can use. All of these glamorous ladies visit, and I walk around looking like an unwashed scrub woman! Strangely enough, I don't care. Then, when Lucy, Doug and I are knocking back the scotch in the caravan Rex from Mr Kai, who has visited every day, arrives. He had overheard us saying earlier that we weren't going out to dinner, and so brought over a complete Chinese dinner in a carrier bag. There are so many kind people in this world.

David Tebet, Katy's godfather who lives in Beverly Hills, contacted Ron and told him about a friend of his called Dr LeWin who runs the Philadelphia Institute for Human Potential. This is an incredible place that has had miraculous success with coma-arousal, particularly with children. David said he would immediately send us all relevant data on the subject. We will try anything to help bring her out of this dreadful coma.

DAY 10

I went to see the hospital psychiatrist, to try and find out about Katy's chance of total normalcy. He seemed optimistic but said it *will* take time and patience for her to be really better. I'll put up with anything just to get her back. But am I grasping at straws? I ask every visitor how they see her: do they notice any change? isn't she looking great? don't you think she's making progress? My enthusiasm for the progress of this comatose child is unending. And so is Ron's. We regale each other with little anecdotes about her progress. We are consumed by her.

It takes only one and a half minutes to get from our caravan to Katy's bedside. The way I achieve this is by having a small ladder outside a ground-floor window leading into the corridor next to the Intensive Care Unit. Fifteen times a day I scoot out of the trailer, dash the twenty yards to the ladder, climb up, climb down into the hospital—much to the astonishment of assorted visitors—and run another fifty yards to the Children's Ward. It takes Ron four minutes longer as he won't use the ladder, so he has to walk across the back of the grounds until he gets to the proper entrance. Everyone thinks we're mad.

She seems to like the Children's Ward. There is, naturally, a lot of noise. Her eyes were open all day. John and Jan Gold came to visit in the evening. They hadn't seen her since she was in the Intensive Care Unit and were surprised at how much better she looked. She started making tiny little guttural sounds in her throat—rather like Linda Blair in *The Exorcist*. We think it's her vocal cords trying to work. I was very excited by this.

During the evening I sat and watched her and felt very encouraged and optimistic. I prayed, and knew she was going to be fine. Then, suddenly, a good-looking Greek doctor arrives. He has been watching me pray and pleasantly asks me how I think she's doing. I babble on enthusiastically about how well she's progressed—her eyes are open etc. etc. He then says, complacently, "Well you mustn't get too optimistic you know, as the chances are strong that she will have some disability." "What chances?" I ask, my blood freezing, and feeling like a balloon pricked by a pin. "Fifty–fifty," says this stupid cretinous jerk, whom I could have cheerfully murdered on the spot.

"That's not what Mr Illingworth says," I reply as calmly as I can. "Optimism and hope are what keep parents going in situations like this."

I couldn't talk any more as I was almost crying. The sister in charge of the ward asked me what had happened and I told her. I went into the caravan and beat the hell out of it. I hit and punched the walls and the pillows and the bed until my knuckles bled, and screamed my head off with the anger and pent-up frustration of it all. I don't know whether I can go on. I feel desperately weak and helpless. I had to get my anger, pain and frustration out. Ron came back with take-away chicken. We had a row. Terrific. We're under such enormous strain it's understandable, I guess.

DAY 11

A marvellous letter from the Davisons:

> Dear Joan and Ron,
> I did not feel as if I was of much help to you on the phone. I felt as if there was not enough time to think of everything to say.
> First don't you feel guilty about a lot of things. Tracy and I are very close as you and Katy no doubt are but all I could think of when I saw her little body lying there was of me saying "wait a minute," and of her telling me about some birds making a nest in our roof and the mother bird feeding her young and our Tracy was really thrilled. Well I can't remember what I was doing at the time but it was all important to me at the time and I never did go out to look at them.
> It's funny but the things that you found important before, found no meaning when you look at them. When I talked to

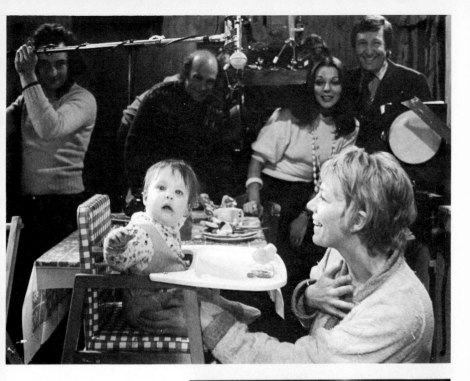

Above: Katy, aged ten months, "starring" in *The Optimists* with Peter Sellers!
Right: Three years old and looking adorable.

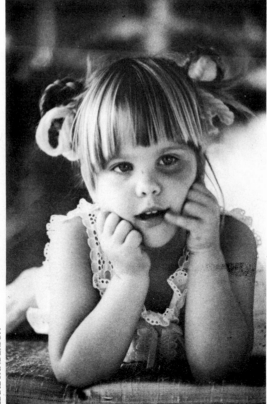

EDDIE SANDERSON

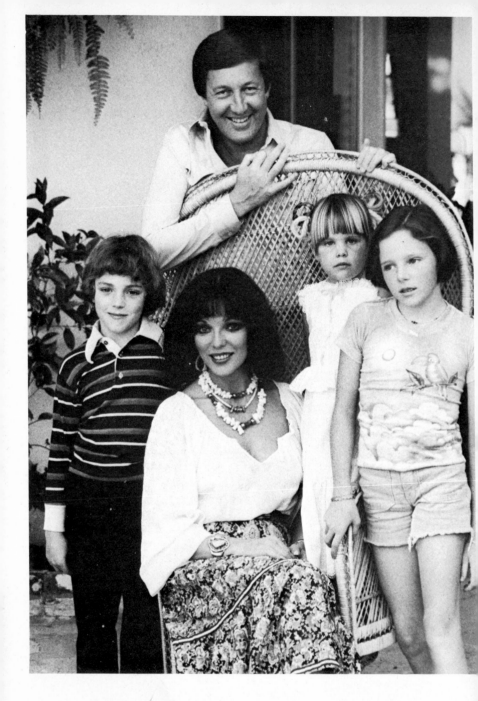

Family occasions. *Above:* Ron and I with, from left, Sacha, Katy
(aged three) and Tara; *opposite:* A celebration on Valentine's Day
with Katy an enchanting five-year-old.

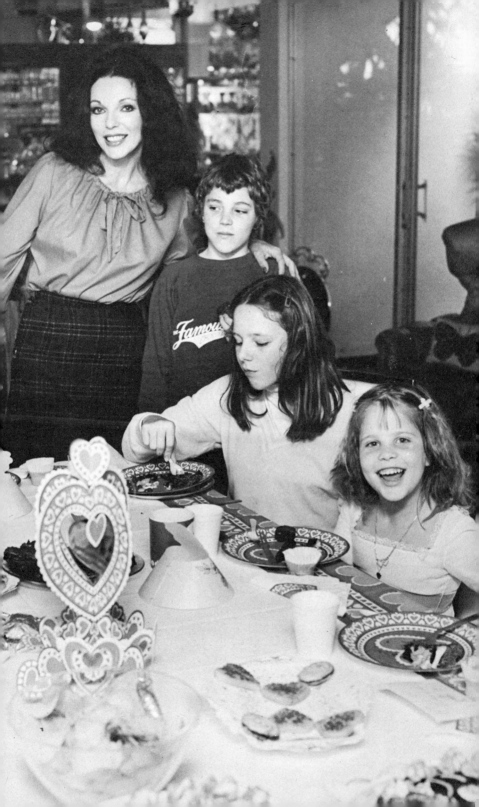

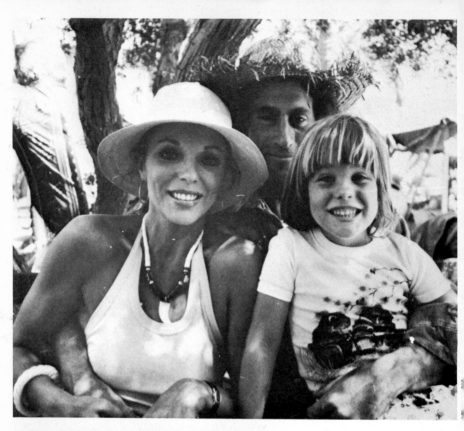

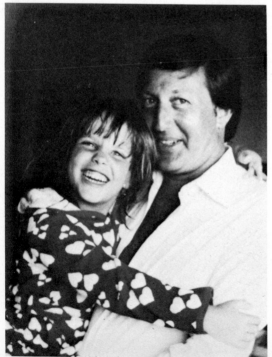

Above: On location in Hawaii
with Paul Michael Glaser
for *Starsky and Hutch*.
Left: Ron with Katy, aged six.

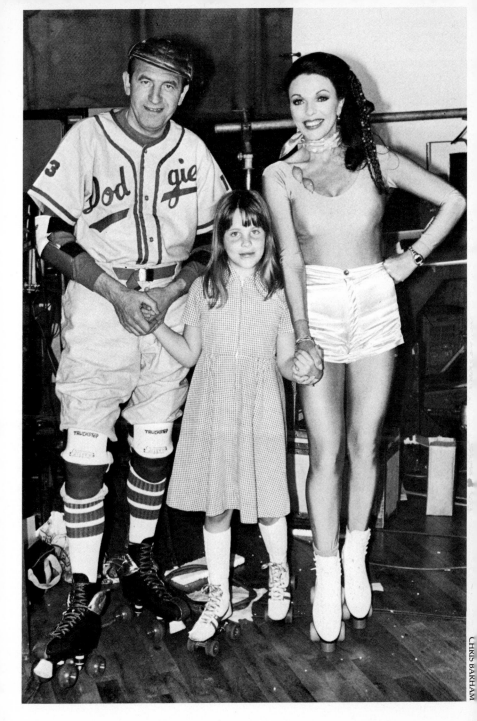

On the set with Leonard Rossiter for a Cinzano commercial.

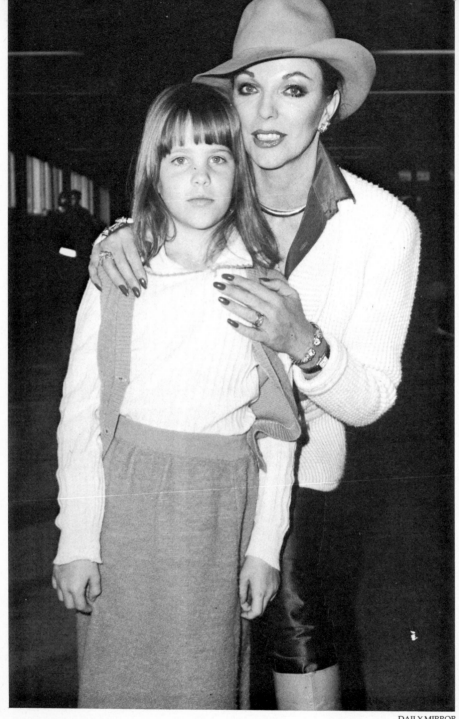

A week before the accident.

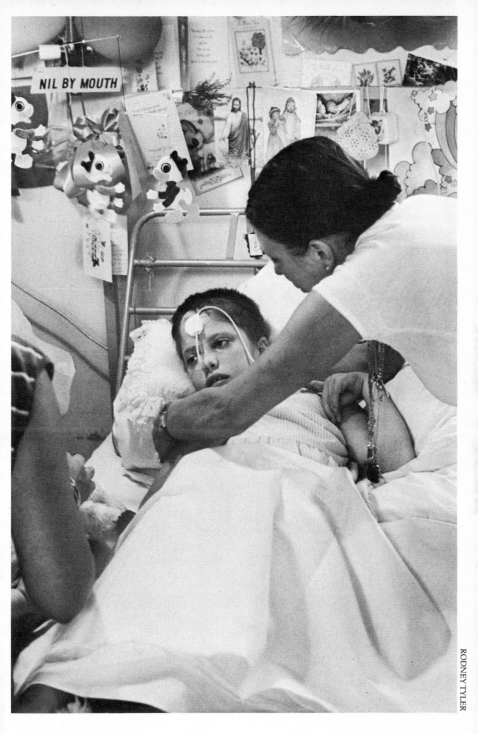

Two weeks after the accident. The photograph says it all.

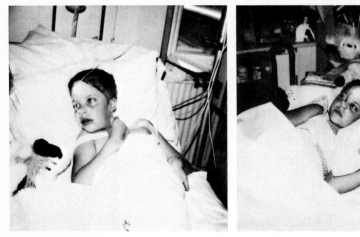

DAY 10

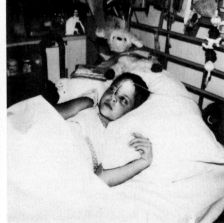

DAY 19

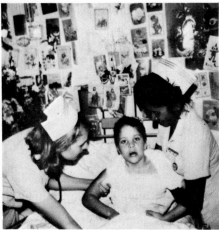

DAY 21

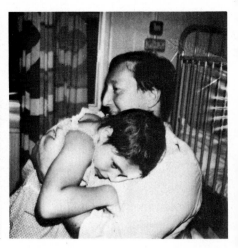

DAY 26

Katy's eyes are open, although she is still in a deep coma.

other mothers at the hospital whose children were in we all felt the same from all walks of life.

I think I'll go through some of the things our Tracy did. I'll try and remember everything from the start.

The first six days in intensive care and two days in the side ward we could do nothing to help apart from talking and playing tapes and things. Then she had four weeks on the ward at Newcastle Hospital.

She was being fed through her nose, then milk build up then they showed us how to do it as you will—it sounds funny but you will be able to do it easy. I used to come to see her through the night but we never used to talk to her at night as we wanted her to get into as normal a routine as possible, then of a morning about half past five to six we used to give her a bed bath with the help of a nurse and I had a tray for her eyes and nose and her mouth and I used to clean her teeth.

She was not doing anything at this time. Then she got that temper I told you about that was a worry. We got that over and she started to fling herself about for two days—she was very agitated sweating and throwing herself about the bed—I thought she could not stand much more, she was tiring herself out so. They gave her something to calm her down and she went back to lying again doing nothing, for a couple of days. By this time we had got a tape of her dancing class music and I asked the physio (who will come to Katy regularly) if when she had her physio we could have her dancing class music played while she done her exercises as they learn that way at dancing, everyone is so pleased to be of any help.

Then she started to put her arms in a funny position and nothing could move them. The physio showed us what we could be doing while we were sitting by her bed, rubbing down to her fingers. It was difficult to get her nightdress on and off so she wore nothing in bed for three and a half weeks. By this time they took the water bag from her and we started to change the bed ourselves. We thought our Tracy would have liked that better. Then one day we were on the ward the Sister said they were going to try our Tracy sitting in the chair. They packed her in with pillows—she could not hold her head at all and her arms in that funny position. Again you feel like screaming but of course you don't, you just help.

Then they said it was time she went in the big bath. Well again it's a worry. I was worried for water going in her tracky* but Alan being there I think a man keeping hold of our Tracy made a big difference, the firmness as he held her in the water and I put a lot of water and made it hot just like she would have had at home and all the time she was in the bath I moved her legs up and down while Alan stood keeping hold of her head and shoulders.

One day when I was washing her face I thought I saw her head move when I touched her. It was ever so slight and then you don't see it again so you wonder "Did I see it?" And everything she ever did was like that, so slow you hardly dare hope. Then they said they were going to try her with a spoonful of water and if she did not make a choking sound her tracky could come out as she was breathing while swallowing. So her tracky came out at four weeks and she made a little crying noise for the first time (it was a sound) something new, another step. The tube was still up her nose but I was able to feed her bits of water and baby foods and she loved ice cream. So she was being fed at five weeks.

Her eyes were starting to open ever so slightly and then wider till they were fully open but we noticed she never blinked or focused on anything.

Her hands and arms were in the spastic position all this time, she was so tight and tense, nothing could move them. It was hard to believe someone so tiny could have that much strength behind her.

They asked us if they could use our Tracy to help students

* Tracheostomy.

by taking photos of the position she was in and by asking lots of questions about her. We said we didn't mind of course.

All this time we got no hope as they said they just did not know what was going to be the outcome. They said they thought her brain had been sheared. In fact they were talking of us coming home with the sucking out machine.

The doctors put it this way. I had said I could not understand how her head had not been split on impact. They said they likened our Tracy to a box of biscuits. They could replace a box (the outer body) but if the biscuits were broken they cannot be put together again! And I had said to them "And you think our Tracy is the broken biscuits," and the doctors just nodded.

When we got back to the room we had a good cry. I think Alan was taking it very badly up till now, then we went down and talked it over and Alan said "She's just got to be all right". So we went to work on her more than what we were already doing (if that was possible.)

They said they had done all they could for her at Newcastle and arranged for us to be moved to Sunderland. I was not looking forward to this at all. But they did everything to pave the way for us. They arranged for me to stay with our Tracy in a little room with two beds and Alan came first thing of a morning.

For the first time I was on my own. I was really scared. I used to sit for hours when she was asleep watching to see if she was still breathing. The first day they took the tube out, there was an old Sister at Sunderland Hospital and the first day there she had a good talk to us (the first time anyone had talked about anything like this to us).

She said to cut visitors as she thought a lot of different faces and voices only confused and she said she would try and go along with anything we wanted as the best pill for anything like this is the parents.

This is six weeks now. We are bathing our Tracy ourselves

and see to her every need all by ourselves. Alan has her on her feet just standing with her feet on the ground. She likes this very much and is very agitated if we put her back to bed and she keeps pushing herself up and down all the time on the bed.

On days when Alan has her standing he lifts one foot, all this time her head is hanging right down.

Next time the physio came Alan said "I'm sure our Tracy wants to walk". The physio said "That's the last thing she'll do, she's got to get her strength back first". Alan said "Well I want you to try her out". So the physio got our Tracy up and she took four steps. The physio said "Well she is moving the right way as her feet went forward and if it was not coming from her brain her legs would have gone sideways or anywhere but forward".

When she was resting which was not very often, we would let no one in to see her. It's very nice of people to come but they are the most important ones (aren't they) and when the body is sleeping it's repairing itself. Her eyes were open more and more now but still no expression. We brought lots of photos and talked of holidays then we asked if we could take her out of the hospital. The doctors said "Ten minutes" but that sister said she trusted us to do what we wanted within reason so we took her home and up to her bedroom. Then we took her to the beach and everywhere and not for very long you know and not all on the same day.

At this time we started her friend coming in every day and taking her with us when we took our Tracy anywhere. When Katy starts to eat she might gobble her food. Our Tracy was eating as if she had not bitten before and she wanted to eat with her hand. Now she uses her knife and fork great.

Our Tracy became very upset when the bed was wet so Alan asked if he could take her to the toilet. They said "Why" when there were plenty of sheets. So one morning Alan carried her to the toilet. I was amazed when she went and that set the pattern. I don't think they believed us at first as they said we'd just hit lucky. So we just carried on from there and used our common sense and did things we thought was best.

One day our Tracy started making a loud noise and her eyes looked wild. We noticed she did this a couple of times after that. Now when we were told the ins and outs of our Tracy's accident they told us sometimes head injuries takes fits on coming round. Well we knew this was not a fit. She just looked scared but we had mentioned this to the doctor when he had done his rounds and one day I saw a box that had been put in her room. It had drugs in and a needle. I asked one of the nurses what it was. It was for to knock our Tracy out. And when the doctor came round again he asked if she had had any more funny turns. So when our Tracy did that again, Alan just put his arms round her ever so tightly and said we loved her very much and she went quiet straight away—now she would not have done that had that been a fit. So what had happened, she had been scared and not being able to talk yet must have wondered what was happening.

When we took her out we took a wheelchair but inside the hospital she just wanted to walk up and down the corridors back and forward, she just wanted to be on her feet all the time. They gave us a little walker but she used to push it away, she wanted to walk on her own. Alan used to walk with our Tracy in front of him both facing forward, his arms under her arms and her feet on his at first. Her head started to come up but it seemed too heavy for her to support and she used to just drop it back (but she'd moved it up) again, something she had not done before, when Alan used to walk her like that I used to walk alongside them keeping her head up.

When we used to take her out in the car I noticed that she was lifting her head sometimes to look out of the window but all this time there was no expression on her face.

That's the hardest part, we thought, not the hard work

but sitting laughing in front of her all the time when what you really felt like doing was screaming. One of our friends came in to see her and he was jumping around the room. Again our Tracy was just staring at him. He started to shadow box and her eyebrows went up, she had not done that before. She broke into a smile. We had to go out of the room for a bit of a cry.

It's funny all the things you take for granted. You would do anything for to be able to see done. I forgot to tell you early on when she was just lying I used to put flowers to her nose and perfume and say "smell this Tracy, it's lovely." One day I saw her nose open ever so slightly. We knew she had heard and was trying. We asked if we could take our Tracy home as we were doing everything for her except for her medicines. We thought hospital was keeping her back now as she was getting more and more disturbed and I did not want anybody reading any more into this than there was.

They said we could take her home for three days and were very good and said if at any time we were worried we could have our room back, day or night.

She fitted back like a glove and now she was home her words flowed back ever so slow at first. She sat at the table, used a fork, went to the toilet all the time, in fact she was really worried all the time in case she wet herself. We are sure she knew when she was lying in a wet bed unconscious. When we went back to the hospital they were really surprised at the remarkable recovery she had made. We asked if we could take her home for good. The doctors did a lot of tests and said she could go home providing we took her back every day for half an hour's physio and we agreed.

Her arm had come down on the right side and her leg was not stiff on the right side and her head seemed to be gaining strength. Alan used to take her to the baths and the beach. We used to let her do everything she wanted; if she wanted a little climb we let her. The doctors would have had a fit had they known. But she was ours and we weren't going to harm her in any way but we were just getting her back to being as normal as possible.

It's twelve weeks I'm up to now. I think I've remembered everything.

Her left arm has come down but she does not use it at all. It seems as if there's not any strength in it although her left leg is great now.

Her sense of humour is back. She was always full of fun and all the way along the line I've been full of doubts and worry in case she's going to be different. We were riding along in the car and I said "Tracy, what is two and two" and she said "five". Anyway I said "Tracy if you do know tell me, as it's got your Mam worried". She burst out laughing and said "Mam, you should know it's four". From six weeks being in a coma I would not have believed she could be like what she is now. Her left arm is great. She uses it all the time, just as much as the other one. She can't straighten her forefinger out on her left hand but the physios said that will come and her speech is getting better every day.

She goes to school in three weeks and I'm pleased for her as she's getting bored now she's got so much energy, but I feel as if I gave into my feelings I would never let her out of my sight again, but of course you can't do that.

She was always very loving and giving kisses and cuddles and I wondered if that would be the same. I need not have worried. She is still the caring little girl she ever was. When she was in Intensive Care one of our friends came through to tell us she had won first prize in the Sunderland Road Safety Competition. So no matter what we tell them it just takes a split second when they are playing to forget everything.

I don't know if you are like me Joan, in the same position. I was thinking all the time if I had not done this, and if I had not done that, this would not have happened. If I had not sent her over the park because it was a lovely day. Thinking that it's safe at the park for them as we live beside a main road, but she was coming back from the park when she ran straight across without looking. I will never forget as long as I live the screech of the brakes, looking out of the window and our little Tracy lying there.

To see her running and laughing with her friends now, I never thought our lives would ever be the same again. But you do go back to living. You have to. Alan is back at work now. He stayed off for nearly three months which is a long time to be off work but they were very good about it. We are just trying to get into some sort of routine again and our Tracy is so well it's hard to believe it was such a short time ago that we were in the same place as you and Ron are now. But you will get over this and when Katy is running in the sunshine you'll both look back and this bad time won't go away but it will be all in the past.

Sometimes when the children are abed and Alan and I talk it's unbelievable so many things can happen in such a short time, and your lives turned upside down. I know it's hard now for you both but when Katy's body is well enough to come round, responding will come very rapid and try and look upon her now as needing a good rest.

Joan when I used to get a bit down I had this story of a little boy who was in a worse way than our Tracy and he, after a lot of work, was all right. Well I was thinking you and Ron might like them and a story of a little girl. Joan and Ron I hope you don't mind me doing this as this is what I would have liked when I was in your position. And when you were saying your prayers I never underestimated the power of prayer and when we prayed I asked for nothing special just to be made strong to bear whatever came. When we used to leave our Tracy's bed I used to whisper in her ear that not only her Dad and me and her brother loved her but Jehovah God protected her all the time. I could not stand to think of her being scared.

Did I tell you we got our Tracy's teacher to tape some school songs. We learned them as well, we used to sit and sing them to her as well.

Well I think I've thought of everything now except to say day or night makes no difference to us if there's anything we can do don't wait to phone.

But everything will be fine, I'm more than sure.

Yours
Dot and Alan Davison

PS Our Tracy said give Katy a kiss from her.

I was so moved and affected by this letter that I wept for an hour in the caravan. But the optimism that Dot exuded from the letter made me dry my tears and vow to help Katy to recover with every ounce of moral and physical strength I possess.

Rabbi Turetsky comes. He thought there was great improvement. They have given her the name *Chaya* when they have a service in the synagogue for her, which means Life. I now cheerfully embrace every religion. Reverend Porter from the Pentecostal Church has visited twice, Reverend Ferman from the Church of England twice. I definitely believe in a supreme being now and will absolutely encourage Katyana to go to church and embrace a faith when she is better. Each post brings more charms, talismans, prayers and crucifixes. I put them all around her bed. Someone has sent me a photo of St Teresa, patron saint of children. It is next to Katy's bed.

She didn't open her eyes so much today, probably tired. Dr Balfour-Lynn comes every day. He is helpful and encouraging, which keeps our spirits up. He saw Katy born so I know he must have strong feelings for her. Everyone has. The letters I receive are staggering in the amount of emotion and care people feel for my little darling.

In the evening I feel I can urge Katy out of her coma with my willpower. We have a long one-to-one session when the ward is quiet, and I think she is relating to me though the signs are tiny. Tessa Kennedy appears. We are both very moved to see each other. I have been beginning to feel despondent. Will Katy ever come out of this coma?—will she recover? I'm so frightened. Tessa is so positive she fills me with confidence. She gives me the *unfailing* prayer to St Anthony, she *knows* absolutely Katy will recover. She has had a Mass said for her recovery and her eight-year-old daughter Milica fasted for one day. I find renewed confidence and faith. Tessa also gives me a medallion of St Anthony and the prayer which I must say as often as I can. I will.

Ron and I go to Lucy and Doug's for a good relaxing dinner. It helps me to go to a friend's house at night. It recharges me after putting everything I have into Katy all day. For an hour or so I try not to think. Ron finds it more difficult to relax, and he usually leaves after an hour and goes back to the hospital to sit at the end of Katy's bed and watch over her.

DAY 12

Barbara Wallace, a friend from RADA who wrote to me about her daughter's similar accident, comes to visit. She is amazed at Katy and says compared to Helen at the same time she looks wonderful. She too feels sure that Katy will pull through with flying colours. I want to feel that, but this waiting is so agonizing and I'm so exhausted. I spend eight or nine hours a day sitting next to her bed and giving her my love and energy. I feel drained. I go to the caravan and try to relax by watching television and putting on make-up for the first time in nearly a fortnight. But then Ron calls—her temperature has risen to 39.8. What the hell does that mean?? I rush over to the ward and Ron and the nurses are covering her body with wet towels to bring the fever down. No one knows what 39.8 is—is it 102,

103—105? How the centigrade thing has messed things up. Katy has apparently developed a bladder infection from the catheter being there for twelve days. We desperately call Lionel. He says this is normal and not to worry—ninety-eight per cent of people with catheters get infections after several days. A very intelligent woman doctor comes to see Katy and is confident and reassuring. We get the temperature down finally and Katy seems to sleep. We go to dinner at Maggie and Rod's. I stay the night in a decent bed for the first time in twelve nights, and have ten hours' sleep, which I desperately need.

The material from the Philadelphia Institute for Human Potential arrived. It is fascinating and we immediately started to put into practice some of the methods that are recommended to arouse Katy. Strangely, some of them we are already doing, for example, having brightly-coloured mobiles and cards and shapes around her to stimulate her visually. There is an intensive therapy involved, in which every hour, regularly for ten hours a day, every aspect of the child's brain is stimulated.

1. Banging two bits of wood together, or something which will make a loud noise to stimulate hearing.

2. Making the child smell things with a strong odour— ammonia, perfume, garlic.

3. Applying slight pressure or pain to the feet and hands, arms and legs, and moving them manually.

4. Stroking parts of the body with things of different textures—e.g. feathers, silk, velvet, even something hard.

5. Putting something strong-tasting on the tongue—e.g. mustard, lemon, honey.

6. Talking and playing tapes of familiar voices and sounds, with the aid of a Sony Walkman and headphones. This, of course, we are already doing.

7. Shining a torch into the eyes. This is particularly good for

Katy to try to get her right pupil, which is still so dilated, to react to the stimulus of light.

We shall do all these things and hope and pray they work.

DAY 13

Nothing much to report. Katy's temperature goes up and down but they have the situation under control. She looks beautiful. The short hair suits her and her colour is good. She has started making more definite loud noises like moans and cow-moos in her throat. She can't control her sweating and her head gets very hot.

It is now nearly two weeks after the accident and I am beginning to be aware of, and to be able to think about, the circumstances of it. Earlier I really didn't want to learn the details. I knew it would only upset me more and do no good in terms of the rehabilitation programme we are working on with her. But for the record I must set it down.

Katy was playing tag with Georgina and her cousin in the garden of Georgina's aunt's house in Ascot. The cousin, a boy aged about eleven—I don't even know his name—got bored and wandered off. The girls got giggly and started to "stalk" him. He opened a broken gate at the bottom of the garden and crossed into a main road. Georgina and Katy, hand in hand, blindly followed him. The car was driven at twenty-seven miles-per-hour in a thirty-mile speed limit by an eighteen-year-old who was taking his father home from a hospital check-up (how ironic!). He was driving carefully and, according to the police and forensic experts who examined the area, the trees, the skid marks, and eye-witnesses, he did all he could to avoid them. But he couldn't. Georgina was thrown and broke her leg in three places. Katy was thrown by the bumper and her head hit the kerb.

A woman in the house opposite appeared almost immediately and wrapped Katy in a blanket while they waited for the police and ambulance. They thought she had just fainted as she didn't seem too badly hurt and Georgina was screaming her head off. Ron discovered all this information. I can only think of it in a matter-of-fact way. To get emotional will only destroy me. If I allow that to happen I am no help to my child.

When the two children were taken by ambulance to Heatherwood Hospital, they discovered that Katy had lapsed into a coma. Her hair was cropped in case she had to have an operation to reduce the swelling in the brain. One of the doctors called the Central Middlesex Hospital for advice as it is one of the top neurosurgical hospitals in Britain and, as luck would have it—and my God there is such good luck here as well as bad—a marvellous doctor from Khartoum happened to be on duty. He persuaded Heatherwood to send Katy there for a brain scan by a new sophisticated machine that gives a kind of X-ray of the brain. The ambulance did the run with Katy in twenty minutes—it normally takes an hour. The attendant and driver have contacted us and Ron has spoken to them. They have been wonderful and they have said that she *never* stopped breathing—a very important sign.

May, a cleaner from the Central Middlesex Hospital, told me she was on duty in the Intensive Care Unit the night they brought Katy in on a stretcher, at about seven o'clock. "I cried when I first saw her," said May. "I've seen many a sad case, but this was so terrible. I knew this beautiful little girl wouldn't live to see the day break, she was in such a bad way."

Well Katy has proved May wrong. She has proved a lot of people wrong, and I know she's going to prove them *all* wrong and recover totally.

DAY 14

Another letter from the Davisons:

Dear Joan and Ron

After I had wrote that long letter I thought I would send you these photos and tell you a bit about them. The one where all the nurses are on is in Newcastle Hospital. It was took five weeks after the accident and as you will be able to see our Tracy's eyes are not open very much and you can see the patch on the right side of her head where the brain probe was put in. She still has the tube in her nose and the plaster on her neck where her Tracky was. Our Tracy loves to dress up so when she came home for a couple of days my sister made her them punk things and for a laugh we dressed her up in them and took a couple of photos and as you can see by her expression she's not back to normal yet by a long way.

Also she could not stand by herself yet and my sister and her boys supported her. Also it started to really bother her about having no hair at this time and she would not look in the mirror at all. But she made us laugh. I told you she always had a great sense of humour. She said to Alan one day "Dad you know when you used to call me Goldilocks, well now you'll have to call me baldylocks." Then there's the one where she's with her best friend, this was taken at about twelve weeks and you can tell by the giggles that she's coming back to us again, so I've got a letter as well here that she got off one of the nurses. After you have seen it and the photos could you pop them back in the envelope I'm sending please as I would like to keep them. You can see the progress is pretty quick once it gets going.

Also they lose a lot of weight but it soon comes back. Our Tracy is about back to normal now.

I hope this has helped a bit.

All the best
Dot and Alan

PS When you feel up to it please let us know how Katy comes on.

A letter came from Pauline Collins and John Alderton, who are having a special Mass said for Katy in the little church near where Mummy is buried. Letters and flowers keep pouring in with messages of hope, faith and cheer. Katy's corner of the ward looks really jolly and colourful. I have put up all her cards and the mobiles which I bought at Selfridges. She is definitely more aware. Mr Illingworth seems pleased. When the physiotherapists sat her up after her session her head remained steady instead of lolling to one side. This means she is supporting it herself. Sometimes she seems to follow us with her eyes. But they are still blank. It's a beautiful day. I lay out on the grass for a while and said Tessa's special prayer to St Anthony and cried. I must stop wallowing in self-pity. Jean Hunnisett and Audrey came to discuss costumes for *The Last of Mrs Cheyney*. They took my mind off Katy for a few minutes. They popped in for a few seconds to see her, and their faces looked stunned and shocked. This upset me but I am never going to let Katy see that. To me she is our beautiful little baby of eight who is going to become our beautiful little *girl* again. I *know* it. Took a couple of Polaroids of her and compared them to the ones of Tracy Davison five weeks after her accident. To me they look the same. Katy is making progress. It is minute, but Ron and I and the nurses can see it. She has started taking notice of the TV cartoons and seemed to watch them in the morning for a while. In the afternoon I played her a tape her riding teacher had made for her and coincidentally at the same time there was horse-riding on the TV. Katy got very excited and hot. I know she was reacting. The physios said they didn't want her to get so excited before her session. But it's *progress*!

I was desperately tired after Daddy and Irene came. Daddy is very brave as he loathes hospitals and I know how much it hurts him to see Katy like this, but to me she looks marvellous. Irene's mother died yesterday so it was brave of her too.

I tried to nap in the caravan. Felt depressed and drained. All my strength and energy goes into Katy when I'm with her. Then Bill and Hazel arrived and cheered me up. They hadn't seen her for a week and Bill couldn't get over the change in her. Good, good.

Went to dinner at John and Jan's. We both felt good and relaxed. The nurses insist we go out and visit friends otherwise we'll go bananas, and that wouldn't help Katy at all. When we came back her temperature was up to 39°. Frightened again. We started mopping her with cold cloths and then a wet ground-sheet. Finally it went down. Fell into bed exhausted but had to take a Valium as I couldn't sleep. Ron stayed up. This morning I visited some of the staff in the Intensive Care Unit. One man said he hadn't thought she would make it when she first arrived. One of the nurses said she thought she would, and she said Ron and I had a lot to do with her progress because of the amount of positive energy we put in.

Ron stayed up with her. There is a sweet male nurse who watches over her all night in the Children's Ward. They all care so much. But he seems to care even more.

DAY 15

Ron left me a note saying he had a most extraordinary night with Katy. A kid in the ward woke up crying and Katy reacted and almost looked as if she herself was crying. He felt an enormous communication with her and felt she understood everything clearly. This morning she seemed fairly peaceful. Mr Illingworth came in cheerily—he's off on leave for three weeks and his colleague Mr Rice Edwards will be taking over during that time. (Mr Rice Edwards, coincidentally, goes to the same exercise class as I do.) Mr Illingworth said he expected to see a vast improvement in her in the next three weeks. So do I. He definitely does not want us to move her to a clinic nearer our home, which we have been discussing. All the staff are rooting for her from the cleaners on up, and they know what good progress she has been making. Took another Polaroid. Maggie and Rod came to visit with baby Rachel. I feel Katy and Rachel will be able to play with each other very soon, although Rachel is only a year old. I am psychologically adapted now (I think) to the idea that when she comes out of this unconscious state it will be like having a little (rather large) baby in terms of learning and reaction. From then on I pray her progress will accelerate rapidly. Katy slept all through the Tylers' visit. How rude! But when she is in these peaceful sleeps I do not like to disturb her. Her temperature still goes up and down a lot. It worries me but we sponge her down.

This afternoon she started moving her right leg! I was so excited. The nurse saw it too and went off and called the sister. They were very impressed and so was I. She also did it on command. When I said, "Katy, move your leg," she did. Later she started moving her *left* leg. She has not moved her legs voluntarily at all since the accident. Her calves have become quite scrawny. However the muscle tone in her arms is terrific since she started moving those in the first few days. Bill and Robin Guild came over and were most impressed. They had seen her at three a.m. on the day after the accident when she looked to all intents and purposes dead, so it must be exciting for them now. She showed off her new leg movement. I felt quite proud! The nurses think that she can have tiny sips of water in a few days, since they feel she has almost got her swallowing reflex back. It's incredible the amount of things the human body has to do. She finally went to the bathroom after they gave her suppositories. The first time in sixteen days. I had been nagging them to do something as I knew she was uncomfortable.

I went to my agent Robin Dalton's for dinner. She told me

that when the Thames Valley Police couldn't reach either us or Daddy, Jackie or her, they called over to Duncan Weldon's house as they know we have a cottage near his, to find out our whereabouts. When he asked the reason he was told about Katy's accident and that the police were treating it as a fatality. My blood literally ran cold.

We discussed what to do about the *Mrs Cheyney* tour. It's a problem. The doctors feel strongly I should be with Katy during her recuperation period, but the Billingham Forum Theatre is building sets and we must play two weeks there. I shall leave that up to them. As much as I know I *should* work, the thing uppermost in my mind is Katy's welfare, and I cannot and will not leave her.

Dropped off some letters at John and Jan's to Jackie and to Ron's parents in Los Angeles since they're going there tomorrow. John was thrilled to hear about Katy's legs moving. There is an international network of friends who repeat news of Katy to other friends. Everyone I know is watching their kids like hawks now. Apparently the boy who drove the car that knocked Katy down is in a terrible state. He is only eighteen and can't sleep at night, having nightmares. I feel very sorry for him and Ron is going to contact him and perhaps have him visit Katy to see her improvement. I can't feel angry with him. It wasn't his fault. I know I have a lot of anger, which comes out sometimes in other ways. I love Katy so much I want to give her only the good parts of me now.

DAY 16

A good day for Katy. She moved her right leg a lot and then her left leg. She is trying so hard. There is really a lot of progress although it seems a little. Maggie and Rod brought Rachel again and took some photos, and when Rachel talked to her she responded a bit. Dr Balfour-Lynn came and was most impressed. He's not seen her since Friday.

I felt dreadful all day—hardly any sleep. Nurses kept telling me to get some rest. Took a massive sleeping pill at 9.30 and zonked out.

DAY 17

I felt great after twelve hours' sleep. Katy had a good night. No change in condition but still moving legs and arms.

Had to do photo for the *Sunday Telegraph Magazine*. Went to London, for hair, make-up etc. Rushed back to hospital. Noree Wilson and her daughter were there with lots of horsey things for Katy to touch and feel—reins, horseshoes and so on. I think she responded a bit. Barbara Wallace came with her nineteen-year-old daughter Helen, who had worse accident a year ago and looks as good as new. Barbara said Katy looks so much better than last Thursday and she talked to her and said this was the same stage Helen was in. Then Martin Rice Edwards, who has taken over while Mr Illingworth is on holiday, arrived. He goes to the same exercise class as me, so I know him. What a small world! He does not seem overly optimistic which deflated us tremendously. We both got very depressed.*

I prayed hard with Katy to St Anthony, and said my own prayers which are to give her my strength and will her to get out of the coma. She will. She must. Then the sister of the kids' ward, who had already prevented me taking a phone call ("Sorry we can't break the rules" type), came over while I was talking to a lovely nurse who was warm and sympathetic and said to me, when I said I thought Katy was looking good, "Oh

* Mr Rice Edwards would like to point out that at that stage it would have been impossible to give an absolute assurance that Katy would make a complete recovery—no experienced neurosurgeon could possibly have said so.

appearances can be deceptive you know." And then added this little gem to really bring me down: "You mustn't be so optimistic." Why do most doctors and some nurses feel optimism is wrong? Hope is all that we have. Optimism and faith are our strength for Katy to pull out of this and be as good as new. Please God.

Ron and I both felt exceedingly depressed. We called Mrs Davison about her Tracy. She was not there, but we spoke to her brother and he told us that they were the same with Tracy. He said that their doctors were total pessimists and never told them what to expect.

DAY 18

Looked awful. My face was puffed up on one side like a balloon, and I'd had very little sleep. Had a crying fit in the morning. Felt very low, and looking at that beautiful unconscious little baby I don't think I can keep up a brave front much longer. But I must and I will. We feel that this hospital is still the best place for her in spite of the fact that a certain amount of bureaucratic red tape has crept into the ward, particularly since the new sister came back from holiday. I didn't get my salad lunch today, which they usually give me as I can't eat cooked food at lunchtime. I don't care at all about eating so the nurses have been coaxing me with salads. I know it is a tiny thing that I didn't get one today but I find it unreasonably upsetting. I seem to overreact to silly minor things and yet remain calm with Katy.

I went to the dentist. He decided he must take out a back tooth that was making my face swollen *immediately*. That's all I need. Then I thought of how brave Katy has been and got on with it. Normally I would never dream of having a tooth out without a general anaesthetic.

At the hospital Tara had arrived back from ten days in the

South of France, staying with Roger and Luisa Moore who looked after her. She was delighted to see the difference in Katy in the eleven days, and gave her a lovely floppy toy dog and me a good luck ivory charm. I think I really need that now.

Between 8.30 and ten p.m. I had a very good one-to-one session with Katy, when we just communicated together. She seems to respond more. She was trying desperately hard to lift her head up from the pillow and did it at least a dozen times. She has immense strength in her shoulders and arms. Muscles like a weightlifter. Her whole body was soaked with sweat and her right pupil dilated a lot with the effort. I feel this is a good sign. Also her legs are now moving a lot and her tongue started sticking out a bit for the first time. When we spray mineral water on her cheek she winces. Every day there are tiny signs of new things. It is slow, I know, but we must be psychologically prepared for a long haul. This is almost like a test, I feel, for the three of us. I must start taking care of myself again. Eating properly, vitamins, even exercising, so I can be as strong and fit as possible to give her every ounce of help. We called Sacha and Robert in California and told them to stay there until 30th August but we must get Fiona (Katy's nanny) back as I have to start rehearsals and we need her to help. Ron brought in Southern Fried Chicken for dinner, which we ate in the caravan. Went back to say goodnight to Katy. She was sleeping very peacefully—and without the feeding tube down her throat! The sister told me she had ripped it out! Clever girl! Every little gesture and movement she makes we hang on to with new hope.

DAY 19

Went in at nine and she was lying awake looking gorgeous. I sat and talked and she started doing her little trick—trying hard to move her shoulders and head off the bed, and she does indeed get them off at least six or eight inches. Doctors came and gave their usual guarded opinions. They do agree that progress is being made but don't give the outcome. Martin Rice Edwards said yesterday, when I was giving Katy a "riding lesson" and making her pull on the reins, "Don't worry, Joan, you'll have her back on a horse soon." Encouraging from him. God, I hope so.

A headmistress from a nearby school who had contacted me about another little girl this had happened to, came over to talk and play some tapes. This little girl came out of the coma in two weeks and obviously wasn't as badly hurt as Katy. There is a child in the ward who screams and cries *all* the time. She dirties her bed, then plays with it, climbs out of her cot and goes over to Katy's bed. I'm worried sick that Katy could get a disease because her resistance is very low now. The constant screaming seems to affect her, too, as she stiffens up whenever she hears the other child yelling. I think I'm starting to crack up. I have to take antibiotics because there is an infection where I had the tooth out, and they always depress me. Anyway, Tara came over. She started a temporary job today with Warwick Records and she brought lots of tapes and talked to Katy. It was good and I think Katy responded to her, in spite of the incessant screaming, which is getting on everyone's nerves. I know I should feel compassion for the poor child, and I do, but it's as much as I can do to keep myself together. When I'm with Katy I do this terrific happy, funny act, and I must keep it going for her even though I feel this crushing misery enveloping me.

Nicky Clinch came over. Katy always liked him even though he's twenty-one and she's only eight, and when he asked her to move her legs for him she did—seven times or more! She is trying desperately hard, my brave darling daughter, to become conscious. Her willpower is magnificent. We all felt good and went to Robin Guild's for dinner and peeked in at Katy at midnight. Sleeping beautifully. Looks like an angel.

DAY 20

Today Katy moved her legs even more and her latest trick is bending the left one, which means that when she can bend both she will be able to sit in a chair! Ron and I were very proud because the physiotherapists said she was so much more relaxed during her session. She has definite periods of real sleeping and semi-consciousness now. I tried giving her a lollypop to lick and asked her to put out her tongue. She put it out a bit, whether on command or as a reflex I don't know, but she seemed to like the lollypop. The other child did nothing but scream and yell all day long. My nerves, which are like Shredded Wheat right now, felt raw. As Katy seems to make more progress Ron and I get more debilitated. Keeping up this happy façade in front of her all the time is very difficult sometimes.

Ron is strong and silent, but I know he is feeling the strain badly now. His sleeping habits have always been erratic but now he can't seem to sleep at all. He paces the corridor outside the Children's Ward, cracks his knuckles a lot and is eating all the wrong things—doughnuts, biscuits, chocolates, coffee. I know I'm not much better but we can't give in to our own weaknesses now.

I lay down in the rest room and had a cry and a cup of tea. It doesn't seem as hopeless as it did three weeks ago, but I keep having visions of Katy the way she was, and although I push them desperately out of my mind they still keep returning and that is very painful. I am trying to be strong but these antibiotics are depressing me. Daphne Clinch arrived in the nick of time and was great. She had a great talk to Katy and Katy did lots of things—raised her head, moved arms and raised legs on command. I am so proud of her.

Went to dinner at Maggie and Rod's and felt completely drained and exhausted. Stayed the night in what Rod calls "the world's most comfortable bed".

DAY 21

It's Saturday. Three weeks since the accident. It seems an eternity and yet somehow has gone quite fast. We seem to have blotted out the ghastly first few days in the Intensive Care Unit and just take each day as it comes, rejoicing in Katy's progress. When I think of her as she was three weeks ago and as she is now I realize how far she's come—and at the same time I realize how far she has to go.

When I got to the hospital today she was looking very alert. Ron was talking to her and she seemed to be listening and reacting. Then her eyelids drooped and she had a little sleep. When she woke she lifted her legs, and Mr Rice Edwards came and actually said, "Well I'm quite impressed!"—that from a neurosurgeon is praise indeed. I don't like to ask the doctors how she is. Ron and I know ourselves by observing her every move that there is a little bit of progress each day, and if we get depressed about how slow it all is we look at the Polaroid photos I have been taking since she came out of Intensive Care. We have sellotaped them in progressive order all over the walls of the caravan, and can see that the difference in only ten days is amazing! But I pray she becomes conscious soon. I played her *Grease* and spent all morning talking and telling her about things she must remember. Trips we made to Australia, Tahiti and other exotic places.

I feel a breakthrough. I feel that consciousness is near but I don't dare hope for too much too soon. I only believe that she will get well. She will, she *must*.

DAY 22

Katy seemed tired today. Maybe too much activity yesterday wore her out somewhat. Nevertheless during the day she did the following positive things: raised arms and legs, sneezed for the first time, ate both her banana-flavoured medicine *and* a quarter of a jar of strawberry yoghurt!!! This is very important because if she can redevelop her swallowing reflex we can then take out the feeding tube. Simon Williams came to visit with his kids but she was too tired to react. During the evening she started to get very restless, moaning and even making a sound that sounded like crying. Then her mouth got twisted in funny shapes and she seemed very distressed. I called Mrs Davison for advice. Dot Davison said it was *exactly* what happened to Tracy, that she started screaming and crying and flailing about as though she was coming back through the animal kingdom. All they could do for her was to hold her and try to calm her and massage her stiff little limbs as much as possible, but the doctors wouldn't give them any help or suggestions about what to do. Dot said that obviously Katy is further ahead in improvement than Tracy was, as Tracy did this in about the fifth week and Katy has just started week four. Week four! I can't believe it. What a way to spend one's carefully planned three-week vacation. The only vacation I will have if *Mrs Cheyney* is successful is after at least five or six months. Sorry about that bit of self-pity creeping in. I find myself filled with fury tonight. Rex—the angel of Chinese Restaurateurs—sent over an immense amount of delicious food. Ron and I ate in the caravan and I started to get angry at the fact that *no one* has written to us or explained to us or apologized as to *why* Katy and Georgina were allowed to play on a main road. It's stupid and futile, I know, to feel such anger and recrimination, but when I think of how precious and wonderful she is, and how much care and concern we have always had for her, it seems even more ghastly. I mean why don't they write and *explain* to me what the kids were doing on the main road? I can't help myself. I know anger is stupid at a time like this, but somebody's carelessness has turned many people's lives upside down—and so nearly brought to an end a precious little eight-year-old's one.

I called Mrs Williams, another one of the parents who we have been in contact with, and she said that her Deluth (who'd had the same accident as Katy at the same age three years ago) thrashed around in her bed for two days when she started to come round. Her eyes were wild and staring and she crouched on all fours like an animal. Mrs Williams said she was like an "autistic bairn"(she's Irish). Well at least we know what we're in for. Ron does a great job of massaging Katy's legs and getting her more relaxed. It's a good job she's strong.

Moyra Fraser visited along with Bill and Tara and we had a sort of cocktail party around Katy's bed with wine and nuts and cheese! I'm sure she would have liked that! She loves parties.

DAY 23

Ron got into the bed in the caravan at seven. He had been up all night with Katy, calming her down and massaging her legs to break the spasms. He said she was irritable and restless and didn't get enough sleep, and he was worried because sleep is when the body heals itself. He suggested I ask for a touch of Valium for her, which I did, but they didn't want her to have Valium and prescribed some other magic potion.

Tara and Bill came to pick me up and we drove to our house in the country. It was good to get away but at the same time I feel this sense of loss when I leave Katy. The house was so full of memories of Katy that I broke down while we were having tea in the garden. I kept on seeing her running down the lawn, riding her bike, picking flowers, gathering raspberries and always laughing. I found a little love note she had written to me last time she was there when I was in Norwich on location. And, of course, there are photos of her everywhere. It was terribly painful and I had to go and have a bit of a cry upstairs and then call Ron at the hospital to see if she was all right. He said she was. Apparently the physiotherapists were so pleased with her that they carried her into the playroom and she sort of lay and half sat in a big bean bag for one and a half hours.

As we drove back to the hospital, I realized what a drag I must be to sixteen-year-old Tara. I tried to make some cheery conversation, but kept seeing lots of pretty eight-year-old girls with long blonde hair walking along the street—and I had such a lump in my throat that it was impossible to talk. I want Katy back—oh, how I want her back.

At the hospital, such excitement! Katy was given some food to eat this morning—mashed potatoes, peas and chicken and she ate some of it. When I arrived the nurse pressed the Dayville strawberry ice cream that Bill had brought into my hand and told me to get on with it. I was nervous that she would choke or inhale it into her lungs but she ate about ten small spoonfuls with relish—almost as though she was discovering her taste buds for the first time. It was really thrilling! Since I've been down in the pits, each new thing that she does is a miracle. I told her I'd been to the country to see her friend Charlotte. I had picked some roses and lavender from the garden, and I put them to her nose and I think she understood and could smell them.

Fiona has arrived back from Los Angeles. I know she is going to be a terrific help. I'm sure Katy will remember her nanny, and Fiona's Scottish accent will get her remembering things. Fiona said that she and the two boys only heard about the accident as they walked into the house in Los Angeles, five minutes after they arrived. Sacha burst into tears and was terribly upset. He and Katy have such good romps together. I can't wait for him to come back but it's better he stays on in LA for a while longer as I have no time—no time for anything except willing Katy well. Fiona sat with Katy while Ron and I went out to dinner with Daddy. Daddy is really upset and trying not to show it. Ron is still being strong. He doesn't talk much, only positive thoughts about Katy. He is a silent sufferer—not like me, who screams and cries and gets it out. I am concerned by his appearance as he's gained a lot of weight and I'm scared that he might have a heart attack or something. He has had more worries than me and I know he has kept from me some of the really pessimistic remarks told to him by the doctors and specialists at the beginning of this ordeal. I cry on his shoulder often and he supports me a *lot*. I don't think many men could give so much. But if you care about someone as much as he cares about Katy, you can move mountains.

Went back to the hospital afterwards, and Katy was very restless. She was moaning and silently crying without tears, thrashing about and seeming as if she wanted to claw out the catheter. I know it's bothering her terribly. They finally gave her some calming medicine and Ron stayed with her while I went home for the first time in three weeks to sleep. I looked at myself in the mirror. God, what a *wreck*. I really looked bad. I haven't combed my hair properly or cared for my skin or bothered about my appearance since this thing happened. And to think I have the *Joan Collins Beauty Book* coming out in six weeks—that's a laugh. I'll probably look ninety-three by then. But as long as Katy is on the mend I really don't care.

Spoke to Ron at the hospital. He is by her side.

DAY 24

Woke at 5.30 feeling nervous. Called hospital. Sister said Katy was fine but I *know* we must get rid of that damn catheter. So what if she wets the bed? I'll change the sheets.

Had to go to Bristol for a TV show I agreed to do months ago. Life has to go on but I feel guilty about leaving her and Ron, but there's wonderful news to send me on my way: Mr Rice Edwards and his colleagues decided to take out the catheter at last! They hope that she will urinate normally and not just have a constant stream coming out. She seemed very sleepy because they gave her a sedative last night as she was restless, and she needed to sleep.

I went to Bristol with the press representative for *Mrs Cheyney*. Tried hard to concentrate on magazines and books in the train but I feel uneasy when I'm out of contact with Katy. I did the usual TV chat show plugging *Mrs Cheyney*. I had specified I would *not* discuss Katy as it would upset me too much and they agreed, but in the end the interviewer said, "And we do hope your little girl gets well soon," and my eyes filled with tears. I called Ron who said she was *still* asleep. At 2.30?? I was worried. That's an awfully long sleep and she had seemed rather dopey this morning.

I arrived at the hospital at six-ish, and Mr Rice Edwards the neurosurgeon was standing next to her bed looking worried. I burst out with, "What's wrong?" Apparently the staff became worried because Katy had slept all day, and so they sent for him, but it was nothing serious—just that she's very susceptible to many drugs, like me. I was so pleased they had decided to remove the catheter. I know it's been driving her crazy.

DAY 25

Another welcome letter from the Davisons.

> Dear Joan and Ron,
> Just a few lines in reply to your very welcome letter and photo of little Katy. She is every bit as bonny as we thought she would be.

Katy

She is the picture of health we are surprised at how much she looks like our Tracy did at six weeks along on her progress although Katy looks a little further on. And Katy's hair looks a lot thicker than our Tracy's did but Katy is very dark, maybe that's it.

Katy does not look as if she's lost any weight where our Tracy went rather thin, although she's back to what she was before now.

It was rather funny when we received your letter, for all our Tracy did know that Katy had her hair cut off as well, it must have meant nothing till she saw the photo then it must have registered home to her that here's someone that looked the same as her, she was thrilled to bits, she said "Katy looks like me with no hair".

Our Tracy is making a card for Katy and when Katy is fully recovered (which won't be very long now the way she looks by her photo) you can show her who it's from.

The ghastly time you and Ron have been going through is nearly at its end and you will start and breathe out again very shortly. We too took what strength we had from "prayer and supplicating" and were able to snatch back our children from a death-like state. I know you'll feel this too that when I hear our Tracy in her room with a friend giggling, dressing up, playing with her dolls and especially when she's just sitting curled up on a chair reading a book, I get a real thrill. When I think of that terrible day and then the days shortly after that when you don't always voice what you are thinking because the thoughts themselves are so awful. Then I look at our Tracy just as you with Katy and my heart is so very full of gratitude and I never thought I could be this thankful for anything.

Our Tracy was always a bright child at school (mind you that side of things never bothered me if they were happy and tried their very best that's all you can ask of any child) but anyway I'll get back to what I was saying. So the other day I had a word with her teacher. She has fitted back like a glove—she is still wobbly a little. But the teacher said she is as bright as a button brain-wise so that side of things is like an added bonus. And I have every confidence that Katy is going to be the same in every way and make a complete recovery.

As we can see by Katy's photo she's more than halfway there now anyway.

I hope the stress and strain of the past few weeks are lifting from you both now a little, if not it will you'll see.

Give Katy a big hug and kiss from us all and she's always in our thoughts as well as our prayers. *Always*

> Best regards
> Dot and Alan

PS. We are not on the phone as I think I told you it's my sister's. She said she must have been at the school when you phoned.

I hope Dot is right about her being halfway there—what is halfway? Katy is adapting very well to not having the catheter and gets very irritable when she wets her bed, which is yet another sign of awareness. She is starting to take little bits of food. Nectarines for breakfast! Every new thing she has attempted she has done so well. Her swallowing reflex is improving and her awareness too. She follows people with her eyes and watches television, although I don't know if she understands it, or if she even sees it.

I had to go to do photos for *Ritz* magazine with Simon Williams. A fashion layout to plug *Mrs Cheyney*. I feel tremendously torn about finally agreeing to start rehearsals for *The Last of Mrs Cheyney* in September. Although originally we were scheduled to start in the middle of August and go on a short provincial tour, all of our doctors and advisers feel that as long as I can spend a large portion of the day with Katy I should try and get on with my life as normally as possible, and

I can contribute more to her wellbeing if I am functioning and working.

I feel a great ambivalence about this. Acting could be construed as a frivolous profession, and Katy's situation couldn't be more serious. But Ron and I have discussed it at length and he feels that for my own sanity I must continue to work. So—the show will go on. And so, apparently, will the publication of my new book.

Leonard did my hair for the photo session and I managed to make myself presentable enough, although I certainly have become a bit chunky around the middle. Too much coffee and wine and not enough exercise. Simon popped in to see Katy and was delighted with her progress—even from three days ago. "She'll definitely be at the first night at the Cambridge," he assured me.

Did the photos and rushed back to hospital. It is boiling hot—got caught in a traffic jam and my patience, for which I am not famed at the best of times, started to crack. Katy had had a good afternoon though, and seemed aware of me when I came in. Several visitors. I spoke to Samantha Eggar and Judy Bryer in Los Angeles. They both sounded very depressed which depressed me. Judy asked if she had brain damage. People, I suppose, think of that as they would cancer. Katy has brain injuries, *not* brain damage and what people don't realize is that with therapy, love, faith and bloody hard work she can, with a bit of luck, be as good as new. And this is what we are going to do. Please God.

DAY 26

Woke at 4.30 and called the hospital. All well, so took a Valium and slept till eight and then rushed to hospital. I always enter the ward on a note of high optimism as I know that transmits to Katy: "Hi, darling, you're looking gorgeous today, what a

super nightie," etc. Today and yesterday have sort of welded
together but they have been great days in terms of progress.
Christopher Gable came at 11.30. He has been visiting a little
girl, Amanda, who has had an incredible wasting disease for
seven or eight months and he has a great bedside manner;
plus I'm sure Katy remembers him from Chichester. We
performed a scene as Mrs Cheyney and Lord Elton for her,
and her eyes went from face to face. She is *definitely* following
things now. Chris thought she was great.

I gave her all her meals. When I say, "Open your mouth,
Katy," she does so, and she eats slowly the things she likes but
refused mashed potatoes (unless it has ketchup on it) and
won't eat cabbage, beans or peas (which she never liked
anyway) but ate all of the yoghurt, ice cream and apples and
meringue.

Dr Balfour-Lynn came and was pleased. Dr Eppel came and
was also pleased. They both feel that as soon as she is
completely out of the unconscious phase we should take her
back home to South Street, even if it means having day and
night nurses, as she will become more stimulated and we can
do much more with her. So this is my aim now: home in her
own environment!—and I pray within three weeks. Please
God let it be so.

Today the physiotherapists let her sit on Ron's lap. They did
it first when I wasn't there and then again when I was. It was
so moving that I couldn't stop crying and had to leave. They
sat her on his knees, legs apart and bent, and now her thin
little body went close to his and her arms went around his neck
and he said, "Come on, Katy, hold your head up, I know you
can do it, yes you can." The sweet little wobbly head with the
cropped hair made the supreme effort, and she lifted her head
for several seconds, then buried it in Ron's shoulder. And
then she *cried*. Real heart-rending sobs, as though she knows
what's going on and she wishes oh so much that she could get

better. She is eight and it is as though she is our baby all over again. But babies learn all the time, and this one will. And *is*.

Had to spend two hours in the caravan with Jean Hunnisett, who is executing my Erté costumes, Fred the wig-maker and Audrey the wardrobe supervisor. Got very edgy and tense. Looking at the Erté designs, I kept thinking: If only I hadn't gone to Paris to meet Erté this would never have happened. Started to get totally furious again about the fact that the people she was with were delinquent in not insisting the kids did *not* go into the road. I know anger is futile and so are "if only's" but I just can't help it.

Jean informs me that my waist and hips are about two inches bigger than they were—not the right look for the svelte Mrs C. I don't really care. It seems unimportant. I feel totally exhausted, even though I know how much Katy is improving. Even the doctors who pop in and out look encouraged. I know I should be too, and *am*, but it keeps hitting me how far we've come with her and yet how far we still have to go. But I do need some socko good sleep. I feel drained.

Went to Rod and Maggie's and I didn't change or comb my hair, let alone put on make-up. Toiletries take me away from the energy I want to give Katy. Both Ron and I look like hell. He has existed on egg sandwiches and chocolate since the accident and Ron and Maggie gave us a good talking to. They're right. We *must* take better care of ourselves for Katy's sake. I feel on the verge of a nervous breakdown and my back is killing me from bending over her bed all day long.

Home, bath, pill, sleep, eight hours' bliss. Ron went to the caravan. He still doesn't feel easy not being there. I always find that time away from the hospital gives me some extra stamina to carry on the battle. The caravan is so tiny and restricted after hours at Katy's side, and being able to spend an evening with close friends and then have a good night's sleep in a decent bed is a great tonic. But somehow Ron is never comfortable away from the hospital, and even if he does come out for dinner he finds he has to go after an hour or so and often gets up and leaves in the middle of dinner. He knows the break is beneficial for us and whatever is good for us will be good for Katy, but he just needs to be near her all the time.

Another letter from the Davisons. They have been such an inspiration and so helpful.

Dear Joan and Ron

Hope you are still bearing up considering the situation.

When you were on the phone Joan, I've been thinking about what you were saying about Katy not taking the water. Well she will if she's not already doing so by the time you get this.

I thought I would tell you what we did with our Tracy. Well after the water you graduate to other things and we thought of what we could get that would be of some significance and to create a different sensation after lying asleep and not drinking! We wanted to get things that would stimulate her mouth into moving so we got pure juice with no sugar in, apple, grapefruit, pineapple, orange etc. and we kept hold of a piece of orange and put it to her mouth. We did this a few times and she eventually moved her mouth up and down, as we thought they had a double purpose to stimulate while doing her good at the same time.

Please forgive me for suggesting things if you've already thought of them yourselves but you are both in our thoughts all the time as we know what you are going through.

And don't forget we are at your disposal at any time.

Dot and Alan

DAY 27

Woke at eight feeling good and refreshed. Sent John, our driver, and Fiona out to get goodies for Katy to eat and went to hospital. What a surprise!—she was sitting propped up in an armchair all by herself! She looked rather calm and peaceful until I arrived, and then started reacting when she was aware of me: she moved her head, stiffened her limbs and slumped down in the chair. I know she recognized me but I wonder if she knows I'm Mama?

Played tapes and we had long talks. She listened *so* intently, especially when I told her about our holidays in Greece and Australia and about her friends. I have never talked so much as I have in the past twenty-seven days. She must be sick of my voice, which seems to have become deeper! Ron has set up a video cassette and we play her tapes which she watches. She is always interested in the people cleaning the ward and the staff walking about. I feel very strong today and even look better. Maybe I won't turn into a hag after all. Gave Katy lunch— cottage pie, mashed potato, strawberry mousse and orange squash. She ate it all. She is so brilliant!

Ron told me they had taken her for her first bath, while I was in the caravan. He carried her again and she started to cry. The person who Katy was staying with when she had the accident was there. She must have been sent into shock at the sight of Katy. I didn't see her. I don't really feel I can face her at the moment. Ron looks exhausted and his ankle hurts and is very swollen. Maybe it's because of carrying Katy? She was awake all day and looked properly alert. Didn't nap at all. She listened to tapes and I talked, and then I played the Charlie Brown video cassette. For the first time she really looked like my Katy: the same intent expression she used to have when watching something that interests her on TV.

The physiotherapists worked on her to lift her head while she was sitting up, and I had to help by giving her some food she liked. I gave her chocolate mousse that had been brought for her from Fortnum's. It was a bit like training a puppy! It was quite hard to do as her head still has a tendency to loll and she didn't look all that happy, but she did hold it up for a second or so and the physios were very pleased. I think everyone is falling in love with her—and who can blame them? The nice ladies from the League of Friends pop over regularly and *everyone* asks about her. She looked so good propped up in the pretty nightie that Maggie's mother made, on her pink Porthault pillows and with her head up. She held court for a while with her visitors. I gave her dinner—mashed potatoes, mince and caramel—and she took it all. She was settled down at 8.30 after over twelve hours of *total* wakefulness.

Martin Rice Edwards came and said there was no reason for us not to feel fairly optimistic now. I feel totally optimistic—maybe I shouldn't, but I won't let that enter my mind. We mustn't get complacent. There is a complete rehabilitation programme ahead of us. Months and months. For the first time I feel slightly relaxed, although I know I can hit the pits again. I am trying to act and live as normal a life as possible, if that is possible living in a caravan outside a hospital.

DAY 28

Four weeks today. It doesn't seem possible. Stayed the night in the caravan so got to Katy early. She had been fed and they had discontinued the drip feed but kept the tube down her throat. She was quite sleepy this morning.

She had mince and mash *again* for lunch—hospital food isn't gourmet but we brought in things like yoghurt, Ribena, apple-juice, bananas, chocolate mousse and McDonald's milkshakes to get the food down. I know she will feel so much better when the damn tube is out. Although she started off the day lethargically I managed to rouse her and we ended up having a good old heart-to-heart talk. Her eyes never left my face as I told her stories about our holidays and water-skiing. Our letter to all our friends appeared in *Screen International*. Everyone's been so kind and still cards and letters and presents and flowers arrive each day. She has 185 cards and I've stuck them all up around her bed with Blu-Tack!

All Katy's visitors say her improvement is slow but sure and everyone seems to agree we *must* get her home as soon as we can where she will get better faster. Barbara says that's what happened with Helen. Mr Illingworth returns on 8th September—the same day I start rehearsals—and we're aiming and hoping and praying that at the end of that week he'll allow her home.

Ron's ankles were still painful and swollen so finally he went to Dr Eppel. I had jokingly said it must be gout since his eating habits are *dreadful*. And guess what—it is! Poor darling, it must be so painful. He has to take loads of antibiotics and try and stay off his feet, which will not be easy as Katy loves him to carry her.

I gave Katy a lot of stimulation from six to eight tonight: smells, touch, feel, noise. She reacts sometimes definitely, but oh so subtly! I was depressed because I didn't feel there was that much progress today. She seemed to look at her Snoopy a lot which I have hanging on a rail.

We went to Moyra Fraser for dinner. Several cast members from the Chichester production of *Mrs Cheyney* were there, and everyone was most encouraging and sweet. Ron went back to sleep in the caravan and I braved it alone at home. Got unutterably depressed looking at silver framed photos of Katy. Had terrible screaming crying fit alone. I wish I could be stronger. Everyone says I'm strong, and I know I'm being stupid when I give in to my emotions and start smashing things but I'm not nearly as strong as everyone gives me credit for. Only when I'm alone do I really give in to the fear, the terror and the pain.

DAY 29

Woke at 6.30 feeling lousy with the light and television still on.
When I got to the ward at nine o'clock the sister said Katy had
been rather active in the last hour or so. I went in there and she
was looking all clean and fresh and they'd taken the feeding
tube out—finally. I felt totally elated, and Katy seemed to like
to cuddle today. I got very close and we rubbed noses and I
made her touch my face and I touched hers. Colin Hunt came,
and when I turned to talk to him Katy put her arm up as if to
keep me next to her. She was sitting in a chair but didn't seem
too happy about it. I played her flute to her, then Ron picked
her up and we took her outside on to the patio. The sun was
out and she seemed startled by it. She nuzzled up to Ron and
seemed cuddly. She looked so pale and frail.

Sacha and Robert arrived from Los Angeles. Sacha looked
marvellous—all tanned and terrific. They were both choked
up when they saw Katy, though to me she looks a hundred per
cent better than four weeks ago, but I realize that for her
teenaged brothers it's a shock even though I had prepared
them. Everyone I see is either just going to or coming back
from holidays—how I envy them. I look like a white slug.

The boy who was driving the car which hit Katy came with
his mother. Ron saw them—I couldn't. He said they were
encouraged to see how well she was doing and Ron said that
they were extremely nice, intelligent and concerned people.

This afternoon Jon Pertwee came over and put on his
Worzel Gummidge act. Katy's eyes opened wide when she
saw him—it really *was* a look of surprise as he was always her
television favourite. He talked to her for forty-five minutes
and sang and played his *Worzel* record, and I feel that she
couldn't believe it. She has a new trick now of looking at
someone who's talking and then turning away and giving a
little shake of her head as though she can't quite believe what's

71

happening. All the children in the ward gathered round to watch Worzel. It was quite a party! Rod and Maggie and Rachel came and Katy played with Rachel a bit. She was very tired by six and went peacefully to sleep. She can move the top part of her body by herself occasionally now, so I'm terrified in case the rails on the bed aren't put up while the nurses' backs are turned and she falls out. Ghastly thoughts keep flitting through my mind: Will she ever talk again?—Will she walk again? I banish these as much as I can because they are negative. Only positivity must come into our lives now.

Took all the kids to Mr Kai's restaurant. Ron explained all of what has happened to Katy plus what brain-stem damage means in detail. He is very good at this since he has been reading extensively all about it. It rather put me off my food though, but I managed two or three kirs. I fell asleep in front of the TV at home. I was happy to be with my other children and for a few hours I actually almost forgot hospital life and became a human being again.

DAY 30

September. I can't believe it. This routine of hospital life seems all that I have ever known. The weather is so beautiful that after Katy had a physiotherapy session with Sheila and Sandy, in which she *stood up* with feet flat on the ground, they put her in a chair and sat her out on the patio. It was hot and we had to put one of my sun visors on her to shield her from the sun. She looked so sweet and cute, like a Raggedy Anne doll. She seemed to tense when she heard the sound of lorries braking—I wonder if she remembers the accident?

Then Ron carried her around the ward, which she loved, and an expression like a smile came on her face. We took her into the playroom and showed her the rocking horse which received a sort of intent stare. She always wanted a rocking

horse and we are going to get her one. The young Greek
doctor who recently told me not to be too optimistic actually
said that she was doing very well and that they were surprised
how far she had come in four weeks. "She's a very determined
person," said I. "Like her mother," said he. She eats well and
is now learning the difference between swallowing food and
liquid.

We had dinner at home with Tara and Sacha, Daddy, Bill
and Robert—the whole family. Fiona cooked—she is a real
treasure. Sacha adores Katy and kept asking when she would
be *completely* better as he doesn't want to set a deadline for
himself and then be disappointed. He asked if it would be by
Christmas or by her ninth birthday next June. We feel strongly
that she will be much, much better by Christmas. I would like
to say confidently that she will be a hundred per cent, but I
don't know if I should tempt fate by saying that.

Everyone seemed rather gloomy, although Ron and I feel
great today. Katy's improvement is like a tortoise climbing up
the side of a mountain—slow but sure.

DAY 31

Because there have been so many enquiries from the press and
public, the hospital decided to issue a bulletin saying that Katy
was out of the coma although still in bed, so all the papers had
bits about her, and of course everyone thinks she's sitting up
in bed with a big smile saying, "Mummy" and playing with
dolls. People don't understand this process. I mean she had a
serious, *serious* accident, and it is going to take endless
patience and strength from all of us to get her completely
recovered. I feel despondent when I look at her face—so
beautiful and calm and sort of expressionless—though she
does look alert sometimes, and she cries when in pain, especially during the physiotherapy. I can't bear to watch her then,

though I steel myself to. It seems fearfully painful even though it's doing her good.

This whole thing is a nightmare. Every day I walk through the hospital corridors and hear the whispers, "There's Joan Collins. Her child is very ill," and everyone stares, and I try to keep myself relatively healthy in mind and body to face each new day with Katy. I called Barbara Wallace and had a good weep. I asked her if Helen had been the same and she said yes and how incredibly upsetting and ghastly it was. The thing is, when I'm close to Katy we cuddle and I put my cheek to hers and touch her soft skin and punk-rock hair, I feel fine. I feel strong and sure, absolutely positive she's going to come through and come out the same little girl who went in. It's when I'm away that the torment and the agony and the fear and doubt are there.

No visitors today. Several flowers from people who hear she's getting better and lots of presents for her to open when she's better. Had to have a wig-fitting for *Mrs Cheyney*. Went to the gym for the first time to try and lose hospital flab. I'm concerned about Ron's health. He is in agony with his legs and he won't eat properly. He threw a journalist from one of the tackier tabloids out of the ward today. This man had the cheek to come in and stand at the bottom of the bed while I was cuddling Katy to ask for an interview. He said it would make a nice human-interest story! The ward has put up a notice: "All visitors report to Sister."

I'm praying that we will be able to take her home next week. When I say the words "home" and "South Street" to her, she listens intently. I know she can understand. I suppose she is now technically semi-conscious.

DAYS 32 and 33

These two days are a sort of blur. Her progress was quite fractional, although she is slightly more aware each day. As I talk and sing to her I search her face endlessly for signs of recognition. She now can move herself from side to side in bed with enormous effort. She has come a long, long way but I'm greedy and I need to see something new each day. We seem to have taken over the whole ward. There are so many flowers, books, toys, cards, television sets and cassette players—it's total overflow.

I got very upset when we were wheeling her from the upstairs physio room back to the Children's Ward. When the lift stopped, a cranky old porter was bringing out a box of sheets, and when we asked if we could have the lift to go down he was extremely rude and said he was busy and had to go up a floor. When we asked him to please be understanding he almost shoved her wheelchair aside and slammed the gates on the lift so he could use it. I could have killed him. Ron picked Katy up in his arms and carried her down one flight to her bed but it made me so upset I had to go in the loo and cry for ten minutes. My strength seems to be deserting me. I still have it when I'm close to her, but when I'm not I'm a weeping wreck.

I had to have an interview in the Staff Nurses' Room with six or seven television people about my beauty commercial to plug the serialization of *The Joan Collins Beauty Book* in the *Daily Mail* next week. Life continues. I thought I looked horrific and it's a joke I have a book on beauty coming out, but they seemed pleased with my appearance. Maybe I have a picture of Dorian Gray somewhere.

A schoolmate came to visit Katy with her mother and talked about school things, and Katy watched her face most intently. She must hear and I know she must understand and wonder what the hell's going on. Mrs Attwell was most encouraging. She had a son with a fatal disease and he survived five years

75

longer than the doctors predicted because she took him home and *never gave up!* Katy's doctors suggested that we should start thinking about taking her home if we can handle it. The suggestion is to take her on Sunday for the day and see how she does. I'm thrilled. I'm not too thrilled however with the fact that she has been sneezing and coughing a lot and has obviously caught a cold. Another worry. Thank God it's summer.

We are still doing as much of the Philadelphia Institute's stimulus programme as we can. Sometimes I catch the nurses looking at me as though I am totally round the bend, and, of course, the sound of flutes and recorders, and my singing and doing scenes from plays, and the banging of wooden blocks doesn't go down too well with the sister in charge sometimes. But we carry on. I feel guilty I'm not doing enough.

I am staying at South Street most nights because Tara and Sacha are there. Ron's gout is giving him agony but he says he will stay at the caravan until Katy leaves the hospital. If Sunday goes well perhaps she will be allowed out on Tuesday or Wednesday, but I am concerned because of her cold.

DAY 34

Up at eight to do my beauty commercial for the *Daily Mail* serialization. Saw the advance copies of *The Joan Collins Beauty Book* and couldn't really be even slightly excited about something that should be a huge and exciting part of my life. The first night of *Mrs Cheyney* is only twenty-three days away, and I feel quite unconcerned about that too. Thank God I know the part well from Chichester, as my powers of concentration are fairly low right now. Nothing matters except Katy getting better. I mean, how many people in their life get an expensive beauty book printed and how many have a child in hospital with a brain injury? It seems unutterably bizarre. At a time in my career when everything is coming up roses I am depressed, but I will not allow myself to be self-pitying. I just get more determined. Nothing will ever frighten me or intimidate me again, certainly not a book being published or a West End opening night.

The people doing the commercial couldn't have been more charming, solicitous and considerate, and I managed to look okay in spite of an abundance of extra pounds due, no doubt, to the one or two bottles of white wine I knock back each day to kill the pain. I went through it all like a robot, and yet some sort of professionalism came through. The director knows his onions and made it easy for me. I think people are horrified by the experience we're going through. I see tears come to their eyes which they try to hide. I can understand it. When Christopher Gable used to tell me about Amanda, the little girl he visited in hospital who has a ghastly disease, I used to cry and wonder how he could be so matter-of-fact and brave. Now I know.

I had a fitting for the Erté costumes for *Mrs C*. in the caravan. Hated them!!! I think I blame them for Katy's accident. If I had not gone to Paris to meet Erté it might never have happened. Jean and Audrey were shocked. But it's true. Why did I go?—why did I leave her? With all of this, though, I know that the fates *must* smile on us now. She has come through such odds she must come back to us *completely*. She must. Ron has total confidence in Katy's complete recovery. He is so strong and positive and is reading every book, pamphlet and article he can on the subject. Since Aries always get what they want and believe in, I know it's going to happen but I think that I'm still expecting too much too soon. It's the blank look on her face that hurts us so much. Each morning when I go into the ward I want to see just the tiniest flicker, just a glimmer of recognition from Katy—but so far nothing. She doesn't recognize us.

DAY 35

Five weeks today.

One of my weepy days. I felt Katy hadn't progressed at all for days. Got totally manic. Went on the lawn outside the hospital and prayed fervently to St Anthony. It was a beautiful sunny day, the sort of day that Katy should be playing outside, not stuck in a hospital with a brain injury, semi-conscious, immovable and helpless. I'm so helpless myself, and angry, and the pain and agony I am experiencing most of the time I wouldn't wish on anyone. Please God, oh please God, let us see a little bit of improvement. I had hysterics in the caravan and punched the pillow so hard that my hand swelled up for the rest of the day. I feel I might be going mad.

At about 4.30 Katy started getting very restless, tossing and turning a lot and almost irritable and crying. Bill arrived with Johnny Gold, who has been in Los Angeles for three weeks, and saw an *enormous* difference. Well, of course there is from three weeks ago! Ron carried her around the ward and sat her on the rocking chair and showed her the goldfish, but she still seemed angry and very restless. At least her cough seems better and the doctors seem to feel she will be okay to go home for the day tomorrow.

It is Sacha's fifteenth birthday. We went to Trader Vic's and we all toasted Katy's health. Ron went to the synagogue for a special service they're having for her at midnight. I fell apart at 11.30 as usual.

DAY 36

Woke up at six and called the hospital. She'd had a good night. It was another gorgeous day. How beautiful London is in the late summer! Rushed to hospital by 8.30. She was lying in bed with that vacant look on her face watching a Charlie Brown tape which seemed to interest her vaguely. I blew her some soap bubbles, which she looked at and followed very well with her eyes. We talked. She seemed to listen and hear everything. I think she has a sixth sense.

We are very excited. Barbara arrived promptly at eleven o'clock. A nurse came with us. Ron carried Katy out to the patio of the kids' ward and into the car. She wore a cute pink nightie with a Snoopy on it that Rory her cousin sent her from Los Angeles and a pair of pink and white tennis socks. It was a boiling hot day, in the high 70s, not a cloud in the sky. She lay on the back seat between Ron and Beverly the nurse quite peacefully, though when we drove down South Street she started looking rather excited and moved her head and body and legs, although not very much animation showed on her face. Ron carried her in and put her in front of the television in the brown suede chair packed with pillows. *Sesame Street* tapes were put on the video and she watched quite interestedly. Everyone clucked and fussed over her and Sam her cat came and sat on her and went to sleep on her lap. She was very relaxed. There were no spasms and she crossed her legs. She had lunch—an omelette and a peach—and then we took her up and lay her on our bed where she used to love to play. She reacted to the room, but it's all so subtle you're not quite sure you've seen it. It's there, though, and then it's gone. We took her to our loo—she fussed a bit at first and then went infinitely better than she does at the hospital—then we *walked* her back to the bedroom! She protested a bit but slowly and painstakingly her little stick legs jerkingly moved—like a little puppet. Ron had to carry her up the flights of stairs and I'm sure his legs hurt him, for she is still over fifty pounds. Then we brought out a cake with fifteen candles for Sacha and sang "Happy Birthday" and she seemed very aware. She ate some cake too—I'm sure she would never stop eating things she liked if we let her. She seemed quite tired and Ron carried her down to the car. She cried as we left South Street. I know she recognized it and wanted to stay.

All in all a most successful day, and I'm sure it did her a lot of good.

DAY 37

Today her tongue came out properly for the first time, and her left arm, which has been very spastic and bent above her head all the time, was much more relaxed. Mr Illingworth came back from his three-week holiday and saw her. He was most impressed by her progress, very optimistic and proud. He showed her to his colleagues, said how loose her limbs were and how she had done better than he had expected. He gave her a complete examination and said that he is confident now she will make a good recovery within six months. This is just the best news I have ever heard, and Ron and I are over the moon. I see so much improvement in her. We still have mountains to climb, but we will do it! Faith, hope, love, hard work, and her, and our total determination to *win*!

At one o'clock I had first read-through at the Cambridge Theatre with the cast of *Mrs Cheyney*. Some of the cast had come from Peter Sellers' memorial service and brought messages of love from lots of people. The read-through went well but I couldn't wait to get back to the hospital. Nigel Patrick, the director, is being very understanding about my rehearsal times and I am working from eleven to four each day so I have time to see Katy morning and evening. However the travelling is a killer.

Georgina and Jane came. Georgina has been discharged from hospital today and was on crutches. She looked as if she was going to cry when she saw Katy, and Katy just stared and stared at her without blinking.

For the first time I feel relaxed and excited. Ron is making extensive plans to rent hospital beds and nurses so we are all fired up to take her home on Saturday. I can't wait! We were so excited we called Jackie and Oscar and Ron's parents in Los Angeles, and Daddy and Bill. I know now that I can cope with the rehearsing and Katy's rehabilitation.

DAY 38

Rushed to hospital at eight. She was asleep but woke up when the nurses started washing her, and when I came in and said "Hi, Katy" she started to cry. I know she recognizes me now. We cuddled and I told her how much we loved her and how she is going *home* in four days. I know she understands but I don't want to upset her so don't talk about it too much. Had to be at the Cambridge Theatre at 10.15 for a press call. The boys were very nice although eager for every harrowing detail and I found myself getting slightly choked up while talking about it. They are all sympathetic, but they are journalists after all. Simon and I went outside and did some happy snaps for them. I know I look awful. Puffed up from too much crying and drinking and lack of sleep.

Rehearsals went well. I'm glad that there are several members in the cast from Chichester whom I know well. When I arrived at hospital Katy stared intently at me for a time as much as to say, "Who are you?" She is going through a terribly restless phase and we can't turn our backs for a second as her legs are wriggling all over the place.

DAYS 39 and 40

These two days mould into one another because of my extremely hectic schedule. Up at seven at South Street, dash to hospital to spend two hours with Katy, dash back into London to the Cambridge Theatre dodging the traffic all the way, rehearse from eleven to four, and then into the car and back to the hospital. Each time I see her she is more and more aware. Her eyes follow me everywhere and her movements are much more definite. In physiotherapy now she keeps her head totally erect and when they wheel her down the corridors she looks around with interest. Her left arm is still behind her head most of the time and the fist tightly clenched. I wonder if it is because she was holding Georgina's hand when the accident happened? Her walking is improving by leaps and bounds. The two physios guide and support her, but she now takes definite steps around the ward. Sometimes she cries (pain or frustration?) but no tears yet. She is getting more and more restless each night. It is as though she *knows* who she is—her face is no longer blank and little bits of expression are showing. I know that face so well now! All the nurses adore her. The ones from the Intensive Care Unit keep popping over at night to visit her and marvel at her progress. I still cannot believe that she was so close to death. It is like a miracle. We have her this far—she can only get better and better now.

Yesterday Ron and I went out for the first time publicly to a charity gala performance of *Oklahoma* in aid of KIDS for handicapped children. I went to the hairdressers, had a manicure, and wore a new dress from John Bates so I felt human again, and at least a reasonable facsimile of J. C. Ron got edgy during *Oklahoma* and left in the interval. After the performance I went to a reception in the bar to meet the actors and people involved, and was presented to Prince and Princess Michael of Kent. It was strange to be in a party atmosphere after so long. Champagne, cigarettes and chit-chat. It was quite fun, but my heart was still in Acton. I cannot *wait* for Saturday when we take her home!

DAY 41

I arrived as they were giving Katy a bed-bath. I bent down and whispered, "You're going home tomorrow, Katy." She started crying from happiness and frustration. She knows she's going home, I'm sure of it. I read to her from her own book of Written Expression that she wrote in school. Such sweet little stories about horses and trips and her going to Chichester to see Mummy's play which is "very good fun and well made"! There was also another story she wrote called "Safety First" about two boys playing cricket near a main road and one ran into the road after a ball and was nearly hit by a car. "And that means you must always be very careful crossing the road," she had finished. I cried—but not in front of her.

The physios came and took her up to the physio room. I went too. They were astonished at how much progress she has made in the last three days. She rolls over when they tell her and gets up on one elbow and almost looks as if she can kneel, but she's not quite up to that yet. Her head is perfect now and she has complete control of it practically all the time. She herself puts her feet one in front of the other when she walks. She is still supported, of course, but she is doing fantastically. When she walks around the ward all the nurses and cleaners get excited and egg her on. The thrill of seeing her walk is so intense and I feel enormously proud. After rehearsals I rushed back and Ron told me Mr Illingworth had been in to see her. She was sitting in a chair in the ward, feet and legs in good position, hands down and head up, and moving and looking everywhere. He looked at her for some time, then went over and knelt in front of her and said, "Katy, put out your tongue," which she did, and then his face broke into a big smile and he said, "She has come a long, long way!" He said the only permanent damage she may have is to the nerve of the right eye, as the pupil is still very dilated. However, we know that she can see and Ron has been researching into the work of the Philadelphia Institute for the Achievement of Human Potential and he says that they will have worked out a special therapy for it.

I packed up all my things in the caravan. God, will I be glad to see the back of that place! It was wonderful of Willie to lend it to us, and it has been a life saver—but I certainly have got weary of my little step-ladder outside the hospital window. I started packing up some of Katy's things too. I won't take the two hundred cards down until tomorrow however. Breda, the nice Irish nurse, came up and said sadly, "Why do they always leave just when they're getting better?" I promised them all we will bring her back to visit when she is walking and talking properly. I have a feeling it's not going to be much later than the end of October. What a great day that will be.

I told Katy again that she was going home tomorrow. I told her "the plans". She always liked to know the plans. She got very excited and started thrashing about the bed and putting her leg over the side. She's started touching her face now. The Philadelphia Institute paper Ron read said that we must now put the spoon in her hand and guide it to her mouth when feeding her. We have done this for only one day and already she's moving her hand.

The neurosurgical registrar who first saw her when she arrived came to see her and say goodbye. It was he who told them at Heatherwood Hospital to send her in and, with Mr Illingworth, was instrumental in saving her life. I told him how grateful I was and he said that it was only his duty. I have never met so many wonderful selfless people as I have in this hospital, not to mention the letters of faith and encouragement which still pour in. I got a letter from the Davisons. "Our Tracy" has just started school. She told me that before Tracy could talk she remembered her mother asking questions and she felt badly about not being able to reply. Mrs Davison has been unbelievably helpful. I hope we can help other parents as she has helped us.

I sat with Katy till she went to sleep. She was still very restless. Then we went to Maggie and Rod's for dinner. Ron went back to the hospital, too excited to sleep I think. I went to South Street to prepare her room. It looks sweet: Ron bought a hospital bed and cute Snoopy sheets, and I put her new stuffed toys around and all her old favourites. As I walked out I saw her little notice-board. On it she had written: "On Monday I go to America!" Got into bed and had a damn good cry.

Dear Joan and Ron

Thanks ever so much for the lovely letter you sent it was so very thoughtful under the circumstances.

I've left it till now to answer as I know your time will be very precious and spent with Katy.

We are very pleased she's coming on and I'm sure she'll thrive now and go from strength to strength. As well as this being a productive time for you both I'm sure you are finding it the most tiring as we did also. Our Tracy could not be left for one minute and she was on the go all the time but did not seem to tire out at all. I don't know if Katy is the same but our Tracy seemed over-active. Her behaviour also was very unnatural but she has told us a lot of things that were going on around her at that time. For instance which medicine she preferred and I took her into the baby ward and got no reaction at all, the other day she told me she remembered that and I had forgotten all about it.

Our Tracy also said she heard me ask her things but she said I could not do anything about it. Our Tracy started school on Monday. I was dreading it but I know it's the best for her. I spoke to her teacher today and she said apart from her hand being very unsteady and her being slow at writing she said she's sure our Tracy will be the same as ever by the end of term and I'm just as sure it will be the same with Katy. You are both in our thoughts all the time and give Katy a kiss from us.

Our Tracy sends her love.

Yours any time
Dot and Alan

Dear Aunty Joan and Uncle Ron

I could not swim when I first came out of hospital and I can again. I started this week. When my mum was on the phone to you I asked her to tell you that I say my prayers for Katy and my mum forgot to tell you. I am very very careful now on the roads.

Katy will be too when she is well again. Give Katy a big big kiss and tell her who its from.

I'll close now because my hands hurt when I write.

Lots of love
Tracy

DAY 42. 6 weeks. *Saturday 13th September*
GOING HOME DAY!

So excited woke up at seven. Fiona and I did some more organizing in her room.

At the hospital she was sitting in bed watching TV. Very alert. I told her, "Katy, today's the day—we're going home, we're going home, my darling, to South Street." And she *smiled*! I burst into tears and hugged her—it was a definite and absolute smile. The first one! A ray of sunshine. I have never been so moved. I told her we had to take down all her cards and pack up because the car was coming at eleven. She understood! I showed her the cards as I took them down, and she looked interested. I felt quite tearful about leaving. It's the end of a chapter. A terrible, tragic chapter but also one of great achievement.

Carole, a staff nurse, came with us in the car and all the other nurses came outside the ward and waved goodbye. It was sad, but tremendously exciting. Katy sat up in the back of the car *all the way*. What a difference from last Sunday! She looked out of the window and as we came close to South Street her body stiffened and she recognized it. Ron said it is like bringing a new baby home. It is. But this baby will grow to eight years old in six months I hope.

She cried (without tears) as Ron carried her up the stairs. Everyone clambered around and we sat her on the bean bag in the living room and put on *Sesame Street*. She reacted—and then her left hand, which has been tightly clenched for six weeks, *relaxed*! It was quite extraordinary. It went from stiff to normal just like that. Then Annie, the new day nurse we have, and I took her to her own loo after Ron had carried her up the four flights (his poor legs!) and she went. And then she walked with our help into her bedroom, looking around with interest. She was exhausted. It must be an enormously traumatic experience for her but a thrilling one nevertheless. Deep in her subconscious mind she knows that she is home, back where she belongs and surrounded by people who love her.

Tara was thrilled with her and thinks she is incredible. Yes, she certainly is. I am so excited about all the new things she has yet to do. She sat in a chair in her room watching horse-racing on television while I gave her her lunch. And *again*, after, she indicated she wanted to go to the loo. Then the two new physiotherapists, Debbie and Sara, arrived. Katy was not too pleased to see yet another two new faces and was quite stubborn about doing what they wanted, like rolling over on a mat each side. But her walking is improving tremendously and she even took two steps *backwards*—a big step, so to speak.

At seven o'clock the night nurse, Claire, came on. Katy seemed cross to see yet *another* new face and I realize it is rather disorientating for her, but it is necessary for a week or so as Ron and I must get some proper rest at night—and, my God, *Mrs Cheyney* opens in two weeks. At about 7.30 Ron came down and told me she was very restless and trying hard to talk—no sounds come out but her tongue pops out a lot. When he said, "Do you want Mummy?" she stared at him intently with a look that said "Yes." I went up and spoke to her and sang to her and she calmed down. She finally went into a good sleep at eight o'clock. Both Dr Balfour-Lynn and Dr Eppel came to see her and were extremely enthused about her.

DAY 43

Woke at nine. Katy was asleep. Claire said she'd had a good night and only woke up twice when she was wet. When Debbie, the physio, came in the room I said, "Katy, here's the nice lady who's going to do your exercises with you." She went mad! Started stiffening up and making her angry furious moaning grunts and cries, and she obviously did *not* want to do physiotherapy today. However she finally did well. Debbie was pleased and said she was a hundred per cent better than yesterday. I wonder why she doesn't like the physiotherapy?

Bill came over and carried her the one flight down into our bedroom. She was very relaxed and she lay on our bed, which she always liked to do, and looked around, then rolled over twice, propped herself up on her elbow and looked at herself in the mirrored headboard. I thought she might cry as this is the first time she's seen herself with short hair and it could be a shock, but I told her how pretty she is and she took a good look. She did this new trick several times during the day. After lunch Bill carried her down to the ground floor as Ron is feeling dreadful—due to gout (recurrence of) and delayed reaction plus no sleep for two nights. All of us, including Tara, put her in her wheelchair and took her for a little walk around the small park in the square where we fed the pigeons. She didn't react much and just looked at the pigeons, but it's probably a lot for her to assimilate all at once. We stayed out for twenty minutes and then she spent the rest of the afternoon watching a movie on TV with Tara and me.

Several photographers and journalists called and came by the house. They are anxious to get a photo of Katy but we absolutely forbid it until she is much better.

I realize now that nurses do just that—nurse. They do not cook or wash clothes or dust or tidy the room or empty the waste-paper basket. What we really need is a cook, as Fiona and I do all the cooking and cleaning and spend a great deal of time running up and down stairs with trays. Since our house has four storeys, this is pretty hard on the legs.

Also a great deal of organizing had to be done in Katy's room. We took out her bunk beds and she has a children's hospital bed in the centre of her room, and arranging her toys, flowers (which have started arriving again) and the TV and tape machine keep me pretty busy. Still she was *really* happy to be home.

DAY 44

Today she smiled at Annie when she first saw her. We gave her a bubble bath during which time I almost broke my back. I can imagine myself at the first night of *Mrs Cheyney* hobbling around with a slipped disc.

John, our driver, carried her into our bedroom and we put her into our bed, propped up with cushions. Ron and I started having a crazy conversation about someone not having flushed the loo and there were things floating around in it—and Katy *laughed*! A real throaty chuckle. She seemed to totally comprehend our conversation and enjoyed it. Ron and I went into shock and delirious pleasure and played the scene up like mad—exaggerating and being frightfully rude—and she laughed and laughed, real sounds came out of her throat, and a huge big grin. My God, what an unbelievably thrilling moment! Ron and I had to turn away from her, our eyes brimming with tears. It means that not only does she totally *comprehend* everything but that she has a sense of humour too. Eight-year-olds always like lavatory humour and it's apt that that's her first proper laugh. I was thrilled and rushed off to rehearsals to relay the good news to everyone. They were all delighted and Simon says he is going to come over and tell her some bums and knickers jokes.

When I got home she was doing physio, sitting in a chair without arms, perfectly straight, no pillows propping her up and holding wonderful balance. What a darling clever creature she is! We carried her to the living room and Romla, with whom she goes to Brownies, and her mother, came for tea. Vivienne Ventura came too and said she was a different child from the one she had seen last week. Katy tried to talk to Romla—her tongue and lips moved but no sounds yet. It's all right. We can wait. She's doing so wonderfully well.

DAYS 45 and 46

Two days of fantastic improvement. Her sense of humour has definitely arrived in force. Katy laughs often and at all sorts of things—jokes or funny hats or animal noises. Sam the cat is a big laugh-getter. She balances now on a straight chair, can get up on her knees, raises her bottom and of course her head is straight *all* the time. When her food is put into a spoon she raises it to her mouth herself. Visitors tire her slightly and we've cut down so we don't have too many at once.

The similarity between the pride new parents take in their first-born and ours at Katy's each new effort is extraordinary. Today (day 46), I dressed her in a yellow skirt, yellow T-shirt with New York City written on it and yellow socks, and we took some wonderful Polaroids of her smiling and laughing, which Ron sent to his parents. I just can't get over the improvement. She seems so together and aware. Bill came over for tea and we squirted crazy foam at each other and she yelled with laughter. At bedtime I sang to her and read her the mail, which is still arriving in droves. One was addressed to Katy Collins Kass! I told her that and she thought it was terribly funny. When I sing to her and talk to her gently she never takes her eyes from my face.

Mr Illingworth came to see her this evening and thought she was doing splendidly. He says that he thinks her talking will come back very very soon, maybe within two weeks. I can't wait, but everything she does is so magical. She now uses the toilet every time, even at night.

DAY 47

Nurse Annie is off this morning so Claire carried her into our room after I'd dressed her. She lay on our bed for a while watching the cat and laughing, and when he went out on the balcony she suddenly got up on one elbow, raised her body and got her legs over to the edge of the bed and tried to get off the bed. I dashed across the room and walked her over to the balcony where she sat in front of me on the carpet and we watched Sam eat the plants. Then Sam became stroppy and started to attack our feet, so I got Ron to put her into a chair next to my dressing-table, and she watched a TV programme about horses. After half an hour she made a move as though she wanted to get off the chair and we put her back in bed. As I was leaving for rehearsal I waved goodbye to her and she waved back. It was divine. I didn't want to leave. She waved and laughed and looked terribly happy.

Last night Ron and I sat at dinner in Harry's Bar and talked about the horror of the last seven weeks, and what we would have done and if we could have coped had she died. The thought was too oppressive and horrible to contemplate. He said he thought he would have gone totally to pieces, and I said I thought I might have taken a bottle of pills and just ended it all. I probably wouldn't have because of Tara and Sacha, but it would have been a tragedy from which neither of us could ever have recovered. Ron wrote a letter to Mr Illingworth saying how we would never be able to thank him enough. He did not just save one life, he saved three!

DAY 48

Felt exhausted having gone to the first night of *Rattle of a Simple Man* and had rather too much champagne at the party at the Garrick afterwards. Katy gave a big smile when she saw me. She was using the spoon herself and putting muesli cereal in her mouth. Her chewing is very good now. We gave her a bath, which is always slightly difficult, and while we were weighing her (64 pounds—four pounds more than about three months ago but I'm sure at 4 foot 3½ inches she is much taller too) she stubbed her toe and started to cry. I was glad in a way because she had been so docile and smiling since Monday that I was worried—I don't exactly know why but I suppose I wanted to see some of the old Katy grit and temper. Still no tears, though.

Worked all day—rushed home at six after rehearsals for *Mrs Cheyney* and recording *Give Us A Clue* for television. Katy was tired but pleased to see me. Tessa and Milica came over for an hour. Tessa hadn't seen her for ten days and was thrilled by her new awareness and Milica wants to come to visit every day. Tessa has still not had a drink nor I any chocolates. That was our vow until Katy is completely better. She blew some soap bubbles and Katy caught them on her hand and laughed and was serene and majestic. Rod and Maggie came to dinner and they saw enormous progress too. But she *still* hasn't uttered a word.

DAY 49

I'm lying in bed now with Katy at our house in the country. She is such wonderful *fun* to be with and has achieved so much in the past two days that it seems like a miracle. Every hour she does something new. She is now trying to open an envelope and doing really well at it—her hand co-ordination is much better. She can read. We test her by asking her to point to words, which she does. Tara has been doing all sorts of things with her. When she was teaching her to blow bubbles Katy did blowing actions; Tara made her take a pen and draw, she made her blow a flute and one small note came out. When Katy arrived at the house she walked for the first time in shoes—we still must support her though—and we sat her on the sofa and she leaned over and pulled up her sock! Then she looked up and laughed. She always liked her long socks to be neat and tightly pulled up. It was a distinctly positive movement.

At lunch she sat at the dining table with us in her wheelchair and had eggs and sausages that I had cooked. We put a spoon into her hand and she tried to spoon up the food but couldn't quite manage it and turned away and started to cry. The sheer frustration of understanding *everything* and not being able to do most things must be ghastly for her. It made me cry too. Our country home had such happy memories of her with long blonde hair running and jumping and playing, but it's foolish and selfish of me to think of that now because we are blessed to have her back and to have the belief that she will recover completely.

Tara has her pointing to numbers, which she does correctly. She asks her to point to the number of legs you have or how many noses and again she does it. She puts up one finger after the other when we count up to ten. We gave her a piece of jigsaw puzzle and she put the bit in the proper place; when we ask her if she likes something she nods yes or shakes her head no, now we can communicate. What a breakthrough at last.

Her little friend Charlotte came over, and we sat Katy in her own room to receive graciously! Charlotte came with a bunch of flowers which Katy took and put up to her nose and smelled, and a small bag of carrots which she also took and she smiled a lot. Daphne Clinch came in the late afternoon, by which time Katy was rather tired and not communicating as much, but she did nod her head a lot when Daphne asked her if she remembered baking biscuits with her and if she wanted to come back and stay at Chichester. Lots of agreeing nods.

Ron barbecued steaks and we all ate together, Katy in her wheelchair. I know that she is enjoying herself now.

WEEK 8

So many new things have happened during the last week it's impossible to list them all. Katy is now acutely aware and very sensitive. On Sunday night at dinner and when she was in bed she cried and looked terribly sad. I think she needed me and not Claire the nurse. I asked her if she wanted me to look after her and she nodded. I told her "the plans" for the week and she was very interested. When she gets sad and frustrated we try to explain to her that she has been ill and in hospital but is going to get completely better, and this seems to relax her. On Monday, too, she was restless and cried when she got into bed. Her little sad face says, Oh what's happening to me? Why can't I talk properly? Why can't I be like I used to be? Again we talk to her very carefully about the fact that she has had an accident but is getting better every day. She listens intently and I think she felt a little happier. I think she's sad inside at the awareness of what's happened but she seems so happy most of the time. She really has a strong character.

She laughs often and has a great sense of humour—she even responds to certain things on TV. When I take Polaroids (and I have taken hundreds) she always looks at the camera and smiles. Her left hand is still in a slightly twisted position although her control of it is better all the time. She loves doing things with Tara, who is wonderful with her. She got out the Scrabble set and had Katy spelling CAT and KATY and pointing to the letters. Katy picked them up, which takes *enormous* concentration and precision, and moved them. My God, we are lucky—so, so lucky.

We are really communicating with her now. We returned from the country early on Monday morning so Tara could get to school and I to rehearsal. Katy sat between Tara and me in the back, and suddenly looked at me with an uncomfortable and sad face. I asked her what was wrong. Did she want to go to the loo? Did she feel sick? She nodded yes and Ron zoomed over to the side of the motorway, and we helped her out and she threw up. Very clever when you consider that one of her girlfriends threw up all over her three months ago, and less than a week ago she couldn't have even begun to tell us what was wrong.

The great improvements continued throughout the week. She now gives a "Gallic shrug" when asked a question she doesn't know; is very definite in nods and shakes of her head; she waves goodbye and blows kisses; she gave me a gorgeous hug and really meant it; she blows out matches, walks up stairs with help, pulls down her dress if it's in an unladylike position. In short she is an angel, so angelic that obviously heaven wanted her but we got her back. I have given her all sorts of intelligence tests. She knows all the colours, numbers and letters and can do some simple maths. I went through her French school book and asked her to point to *la bouche, le nez, les yeux* etc. She was spot on, except my pronunciation is so awful that she got it wrong a couple of times.

Elspeth March arranged for Roald Dahl and Patricia Neal to come over on Wednesday. Patricia had a major stroke fifteen years ago and was virtually unable to speak for many months and for years was quite disabled, but eventually she was even able to go back to acting. Roald, who did most of the talking, said that he thought that Katy seemed to be making remarkable progress and he stressed that we *must* now get more stimulation and learning things for her to do, as brain-injured people can often suffer from chronic boredom. I feel that we are constantly stimulating and playing with her. How much more can we do? Sometimes this task seems insurmountable. Are we doing enough? Are we doing too much?

On Wednesday I had an interview with *Woman* magazine. I thought the interview would be a general one but all they wanted to know about was Katy. I can understand it but it's very difficult trying to keep Katy from being exploited.

That night Tara and Ron and I went to Mr Kai, and Tara suggested that we get Katy a sort of walking chair so that she can start walking more and not be lying propped up in bed so much and treated like an invalid. It's a very good idea and Ron has ordered one for her. I know she is eager to learn and get better, and this should help her with her balance, which is still a bit shaky when she tries to stand up.

We took her to the first dress-rehearsal of *Mrs Cheyney* and gave her the choice of coming in the wheelchair or Daddy carrying her. She opted for Daddy—clever kid. A great fuss was made of her when she arrived in the auditorium with her entourage of John, Annie and Ron, plus cushions and rugs. She smiled and listened intently to the rehearsal, and when we broke for lunch I asked her if she would like to walk on the stage. She nodded yes and we clomped about. She liked my dresses but when I asked her if she preferred the wig I'm

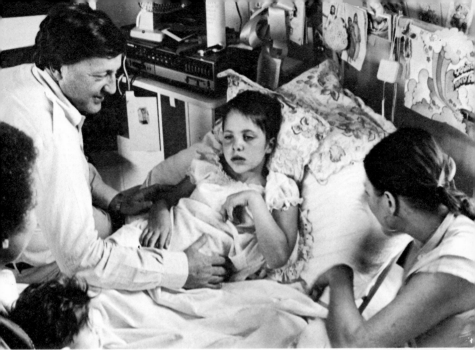

FIVE WEEKS: Katy is now semi-conscious.

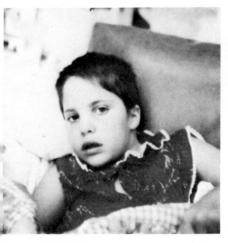

DAY 30: In the sun.

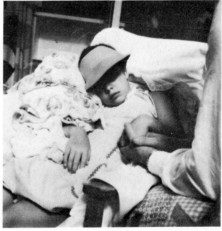

DAY 35

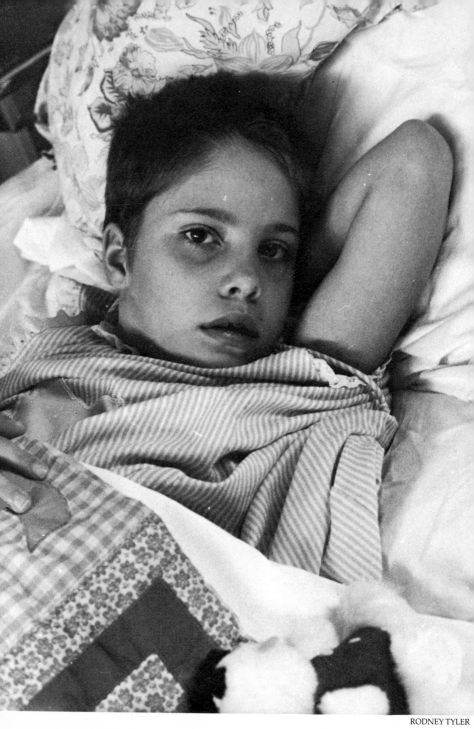

RODNEY TYLER

It is a heartbreaking sight, her left arm is still permanently raised, but she is showing definite signs of improvement.

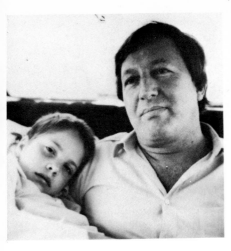

DAY 36: On the way for a trial day at home.

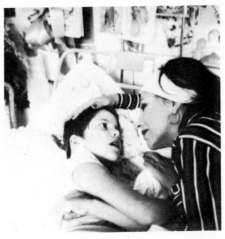

DAY 42: "Today's the day – we're going home my darling."

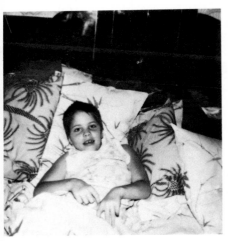

DAY 45: A little smile . . .

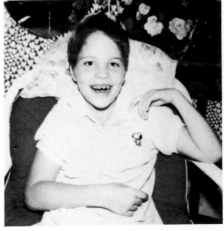

DAY 48: And then a great big one!

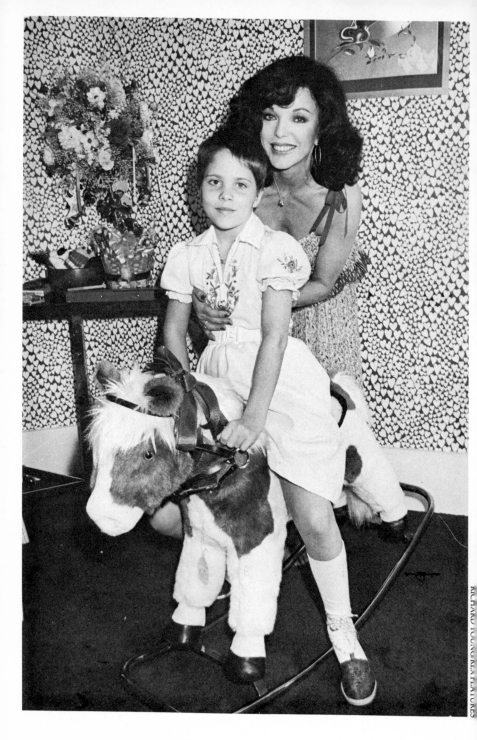

NINE WEEKS: She chose the rocking horse herself . . .

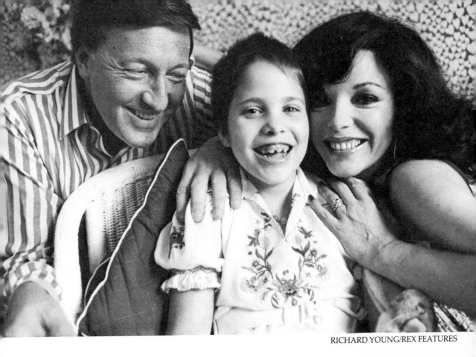

RICHARD YOUNG/REX FEATURES

She has just begun to say a few words . . .

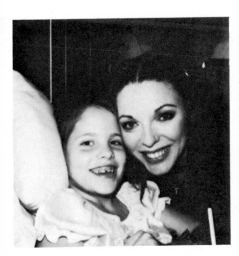

She laughs a lot . . .

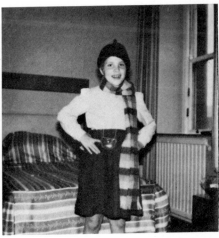

She stands up on her own for the first time!

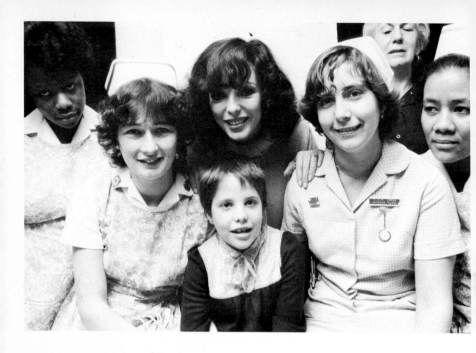

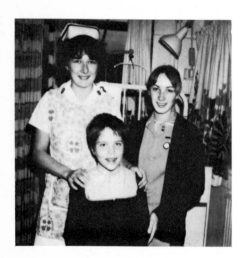

ELEVEN WEEKS: Katy visits hospital – the nurses are thrilled by her progress! *Opposite:* Two months later we presented some equipment to the Premature Baby Unit on behalf of the charity BLISS.

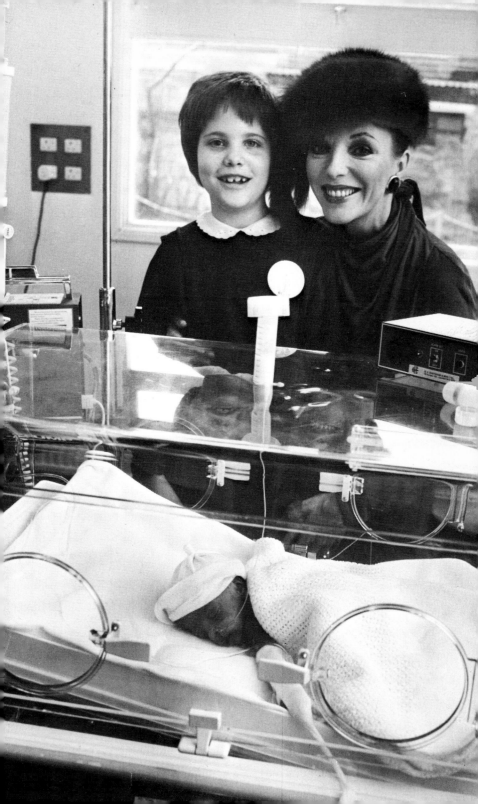

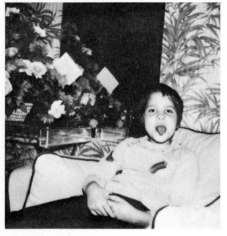

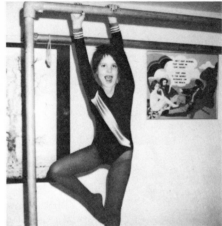

12 WEEKS   **17 WEEKS**

She's getting better all the time!

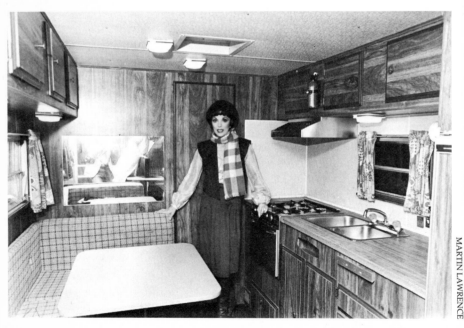

The caravan we lived in for six weeks.

wearing now (a bob) to the one in Chichester (curly) she told me Chichester! Simon and Lucy had bought her a white budgie in a beautiful brass antique cage, and her eyes opened terribly wide when she saw it and she was delighted. We tried to choose names for the budgie. We suggested a few and she nodded and disagreed as she saw fit. I then wrote six names on a piece of paper and she chose the one she wanted—Frankie. When the bird started cheeping she laughed with glee. She left the rehearsal after an hour and a half as she was a little tired. Stimulation is good for her but it can be tiring. We think her eyes are sensitive to light and have had her measured for dark glasses.

When I got back from the rehearsal she was watching television and Annie was blowing bubbles for her. I do wish I could be with her more. I feel sometimes I have to fight everyone off to get time with her alone. I'm up to my neck in rehearsals, there isn't a second free and I resent it. I shall be glad when *Mrs Cheyney* opens and I shall have most days free.

Katy has made the most incredible progress this week, but the most exciting news is that she has finally started to talk! Her first word was "horse shoe" which I could barely hear. But what a step! I was showing her various things and asking her what they were, and she suddenly came out with it. Most of the time it's a faint whisper and she doesn't say much—she'd rather nod than say yes or no—and she seems shy of speaking in front of strangers. But she talks at *last*!

We had promised to take her back to the Intensive Care Unit when she was better, as the staff there have so many "disappointments", and she could be a great encouragement to them. When I told her about visiting the hospital she said, "Mummy, I don't want to go back hospital." I told her about the many visitors she'd had and the presents she'd been given, and she said in a tiny breathy whisper, "Mummy, I don't remember presents hospital." I said I loved her and she

97

replied, "I love you too." So she's putting whole sentences together, which is fantastic because we had thought that when the words came they would come bit by bit. She has to clear her throat a lot, and it's a very teeny little breathy voice, sometimes hard to hear or understand, but it's a *voice*!!!

Katy talks. Ron and I are beside ourselves with joy.

On Friday we took Katy to Fortnum's to buy a rocking horse. The toy department was empty and she sat on three different horses before choosing a thick furry one. Then Ron took her to the Fountain to have a milkshake and all the waitresses remembered her and made a big fuss of her, and she looked glad to be there.

That night we took her to Mr Kai's for dinner. Her first outing! She was very aware of herself. I know she didn't want to make any mistakes. It's not far from South Street, so we wheeled her over to the restaurant. It was a bit traumatic getting her from the wheelchair into a chair. There were quite a few people there and some of the Chinese waiters stared at her a little. But she handled herself beautifully. She drank a Shirley Temple Cocktail and took the three maraschino cherries off the stick with great delicacy. Then she whispered to me that she wanted to go to the loo, so I took her—she pulls her own pants down and up now! After supper we went to Richoux to buy her some chocolates and then went for a short walk down South Audley Street as the weather was so mild.

On Saturday both Mr Illingworth and Dr Eppel came to see her. Mr Illingworth put her through her paces: who's the President of the United States? Who's the Prime Minister of England? She got them right, of course, and Dr Eppel said that he felt she was fifty per cent there. Mr Illingworth said he thought probably more. Either way, Mr Illingworth says it's *very* speedy progress which he feels sure will continue. We must encourage her to talk more since she only talks when she wants something, and also her balance is going to take a long time—although she walks up the stairs three at a time now with Ron or me madly trying to keep up with her, supporting her while she giggles like mad. Her sense of humour is terrific and so is her sense of fun. She got hysterical when Sam the cat tried to attack Dr Balfour-Lynn one day.

I feel she is a third of the way through—if the six-month prognosis is correct. I feel so blessed, especially when I read about the poor boxer in a coma in Los Angeles with brain injuries—he is so obviously not going to pull through. Or if he does he will be a vegetable. It's too ghastly to contemplate.

WEEK 9

Last week Katy talked. This week another major landmark was reached.

On Sunday Richard Young came and took photos of the three of us. Katy looks good now and we hope this will get the newspapers off our backs and they won't try and sneak a shot of her when we go to Brighton. She behaved beautifully and posed for over half an hour on her rocking horse, smiling and laughing and doing all the things Richard asked her to. Then we went to Carole and Dick Leahy's house for lunch. Their two children were very sweet with Katy. She was quiet—as she always is when we visit someone else—but ate the most enormous lunch and had *three* helpings of chocolate cake. And she fed herself.

Then we took her into the pool. Although it is the end of September the day was warm and the pool heated to 82°. Debbie, the physiotherapist, came over and we tried to get Katy to swim but she was too frightened and excited at first. She was laughing so much and swallowed a lot of water the first time, so she wasn't so adventurous the second. After half an hour, which she adored and during which Ron and I froze to death, she was doing quite well and although she was not yet swimming properly she loved it.

On Monday we went to Brighton, as *Mrs Cheyney* was opening there on Tuesday. Annie came with us. Our driver, John, filled the car up with about nine million things for Katy—wheelchair, walker, toys, games, her new rocking horse, special Snoopy sheets. It was so crammed that we had to take the train. Katy walked very well, but stiffly, along the platform with support from Ron and me, and then got tired and asked to be carried, then asked to walk again. She is so proud when she can do things by herself. The suite at the Metropole was excellent, with a view of the sea, and the weather was super. Katy could use her walker in the suite as it was so big, and much easier for her than South Street which has a room on every floor. I had to rush to a dress rehearsal and couldn't even think of being nervous about the opening night.

We went for a long walk along the front on Tuesday morning with Katy in her wheelchair. It really *is* bracing in Brighton! We stopped at a kids' funfair and Katy rode on a little train and seemed delighted. She didn't want to ride on anything else, though we tried. We sat on the beach and she enjoyed looking at the sea and even tried throwing some stones. She was quite good with her right hand but the left hand didn't seem to be able to let go of the stone. She laughed at some teenagers who were swimming and yelling about how freezing the water was. We had lunch in a restaurant and she walked in well, ate her melon with a fork, and sat in a chair with only one cushion behind her back. After lunch I left her with Annie and dashed to the Theatre Royal, where we had a final dress-rehearsal of *Mrs Cheyney* followed by the first night, which seemed to go well. Thank God Katy is getting so much better—it made it easier for me to erase all thoughts of her from my mind during the performance.

On Wednesday Ron and I took her down to the gym in the hotel. We did a few exercises—lying flat on the mat and raising each leg, one leg bent and raising bottom up, on front and raising legs. Then she rode the exercycle and climbed up the gym bars so fast that Ron could barely hold her, and then—she stood up alone! What a great moment! After this she seemed to be braver and more confident every second. We took another walk along the front and she went on the train again, and this time she also wanted to go on the moving ladybird—which she did—and then asked to go on the slide too. We had to draw the line at this. Every day for two months we have been encouraging and even forcing her to do more than she had the day before, and now suddenly she was wanting to do more than even we wanted. It was far too dangerous for her to go on the slide but we were very pleased that she wanted to. I never thought I would be happy refusing to let Katy do something she wanted to do. She stood up alone and that's enough progress for one day. Even for me.

On Thursday she came to the matinée. She hates being in the wheelchair so she walked backstage and Ron put the wheelchair in the stage-right box and she watched the whole show from there. I could see her from the stage and she looked as if she was enjoying it. She came backstage in the interval. Auntie Pauline was there and brought her some cream cakes, and Katy remembered her. She is conversing more and more. Her sentence construction is excellent but her voice is still very faint and hoarse. After the performance she came backstage again. Simon Williams came in and she walked over to him alone! She had been starting to take steps since she stood up alone yesterday. She has to get her balance first but it was wonderful to see. I am so proud of her and she was pleased as punch!

She has had many letters from her schoolmates which she reads, and also one from one of her teachers which was very touching and complimentary to her, and she was obviously proud of this. She looks beautiful, but is worried about her hair and wishes it were still long.

On Friday we went to the gym again. She climbed up the bars like a little monkey, though we had to support her back. She keeps asking questions about the accident: What happened? Why can't she walk well? She asks these questions all the time and when we explain patiently that she was in a long sleep and has to learn how to do things again she listens very intently and with great interest. Her little face is so expressive now. It's wondrous to see.

During the show interval Ron brought me a note that she had written herself:

> Dear Mummy and Daddy
> I love you very much
> Love Katy XXX

The writing was a little shaky and the letters sloped a bit but it is her first writing—another thrill.

What a week! Katy's been doing so much it's hard to keep up. She walks around the suite by herself now. She gets her balance first and her left hand has to stick out for support but it's really good. Her voice is whispery but perfectly clear and we can understand ninety per cent of what she says. She keeps asking about Sam the cat: if he's all right, who's taking care of him and who's giving him food.

She is very anxious to do everything well. We took her to the Chailey Heritage Hospital for Handicapped Children and went swimming. She did quite well, though she was nervous at first. She likes the water but is still not prepared to swim properly. She was such a fabulous strong swimmer before, but I know it will come back. There were two boys about her age there. One was born without arms but he was smiling and swimming and having a wonderful time in the water. Seeing this little boy, so brave and yet so terribly handicapped, I realize again how immensely lucky we have been with Katy. I thought about the boy's parents and the agony they must have gone through when faced with such a deformity at birth. But they coped. They obviously coped well as the boy seems beautifully adjusted. I wondered how we would or could have handled the possibility of Katy being seriously disabled. The thought is too horrifying to contemplate. We must always be thankful for how much God has given us in this amazing progress Katy is making and how lucky we are that she was not more seriously injured.

Tara and Sacha arrived, and her face lit up with joy and she walked over to Sacha and they hugged each other joyfully for a long, long time. Sacha hadn't seen her for a month so he was overwhelmed at the difference.

The week before last she talked, last week she walked alone. But I mustn't get complacent—from now on we must try even harder to consolidate this amazing progress.

WEEK 10

On Sunday all the nurses and Fiona were off and I had no work, thank goodness. *All* my children were there. We had pancakes in the hotel suite for breakfast and then went down to the gym. I wanted Katy to do what she usually does to show Tara and Sacha how brilliant she is now, but for some reason she became upset and started to cry. I think seeing Tara and Sacha makes her realize that she can't do what she used to be able to and it's immensely frustrating. The others were very good with her and told her how good she was at climbing and balance. She has always been such a perfectionist.

We all went for a walk along the front, Katy in her wheel-chair (reluctantly). She does not like to be in the chair but it's hard for her to walk long distances. None of us looked too good, and I was wearing my "Brighton in disguise" outfit. We bumped into a nineteen-year-old girl we knew who had heard of the accident but hadn't seen Katy and didn't know of her extraordinary progress. She was obviously shocked, since the last time she'd seen her she'd been a tanned, laughing, blonde-haired active child, and when she's in the wheelchair it *does* look more serious than it is. I realize that many people must feel pity for Katy and for us. But I don't want anyone to show sorrow. She is a miraculous child: it is only nine weeks since she was at death's door and she is much more than half way back to us, I think.

We went into the amusement arcade on Brighton Pier after we'd had fish and chips in deck chairs on the sea front, and all the kids loved it there. Katy played one of those ghastly games where you keep putting tenpence pieces in a machine and occasionally it gives you a few in return. It was good for her co-ordination and it gave her pleasure.

Tara and Sacha went back to their respective schools after tea and William Hall came to do an interview for *Woman's Own*. Katy met him and they talked. He thought she was amazing and his eyes misted over. He, too, has an eight-year-old girl.

Ron and I are with Katy most of the time so we don't always notice each tiny detail of her day-by-day progress, but it's there, sure enough. Fiona came back on Monday. She hadn't seen Katy for three days and saw *much* improvement in co-ordination (she can tie a bow and almost tie her shoe laces), speech, conversation and balance. I can't wait to show her to everyone at the hospital. We went to the gym a couple of times. She was not as keen as she was last week and kept on and *on* asking, "Why can't I walk properly?" She likes to hear the story of the accident but doesn't seem to remember recent happenings. Mr Illingworth said it is a short-term memory block typical of this sort of case and it will continue for some time. She swam five widths of the pool at Chailey by herself (with armbands), and that is wonderful. She purloined one of my hats, a burgundy wool cap which looks adorable and suits her and covers her lack of hair. She loves Simon Williams to tease her, which he does unmercifully and she giggles. She begged to be allowed to see *Mrs Cheyney* again and we said that if she had a nap she could. She took a nap, though she hates to, and came to the show. It's hard for her at night since she gets tired, but she was walking and talking quite a lot and engrossed in the play. I had to go to London that night for a dentist's appointment the next day. Katy looked sad but not too sad—it was her "actress" look. She is exceedingly expressive.

I had a painful two hours of drilling at the dentist—after which my face swelled up like a beach ball—and arrived back at Brighton Station to be met by Ron and a rather depressed-looking little Katy. Ron said she had missed me a lot and was constantly asking when I would return and where was I and how was Sam? Back at the hotel, we read poetry and sang songs and I tried to get her to develop more strength in her vocal cords. Her voice is still very whispery, but hopefully that will change soon. She keeps saying the same thing over and over: "I'm scared—I don't want to go back to school." We tried to reassure her and told her that she didn't have to go back until she was better, but it didn't seem to ease her mind. She kept asking which class she was in—III or IV. She was in III last term and this term would have been in IV, and she also can't remember whether she is seven or eight. Her birthday was only five weeks before the accident and she probably doesn't remember it, though when I showed her the photos of her party she seemed to remember that. I wish she would stop being so worried about things, but apparently it's natural, particularly with someone of her intelligence. She and Ron walked me down to the lobby when I had to leave for the theatre. The hotel is swarming with Conservatives, as it is their convention and Katy looked for celebrities, particularly Mrs Thatcher. One of the porters said that he thought Katy had made great progress since she'd been at Brighton. It's true.

We have had loads of letters from America, one from a man whose daughter was in a car accident similar to Katy's. She was in hospital for five hundred days and had two brain operations and *still* cannot walk or talk properly. Thank God Katy did not have brain surgery as this is apparently the hardest thing to recover from. On top of that, it has cost this man nearly half a million dollars! We are fortunate in more ways than one. Every day as I see her getting better I thank God for our luck and her stamina.

Each Saturday is an anniversary. It is ten weeks since the accident, about twenty-four days, I suppose, since Katy has been totally conscious. It's miraculous. The change is incredible. Her mind is sharp as a tack. Her humour is back. She teases Ron and me, asking over and over, "When am I going back to school?" and when we say, "You don't have to go back to school," she says, "Never again?" and then puts on a pretend sad face. She's such a little pixie. "No" is figuring rather largely in her vocabulary now. She refuses to eat certain foods, refuses to put on clothes she doesn't like, refuses to do some of the exercises in the gym, and I think it's *wonderful!* To hear her say "No" is a joy. We think she's 75–80 per cent recovered. She showed off today in the lounge of the hotel and walked back and forth swiftly, then turned round twice as though she was doing a modelling job! But she still asks all the time why she can't walk properly. Her left arm still has a life of its own, her legs are a bit wobbly and her shoulders are hunched unless we remind her—but it's astounding. Her speech improves daily—sentence structure and clarity are excellent, but there's still not enough volume. She gets bored easily with things she can't do well (writing, drawing) and it's an effort for her to do them. She says *"No!"* We have to persuade her. She made a card for Tara's seventeenth birthday but it took all Annie's patience to get her to do it. She wanted it to be perfect and became frustrated.

WEEK 11

We came back from Brighton on Sunday, and that night we went to Trader Vic's as it was Tara's birthday. For an hour or two before we went out, Katy seemed very tired and sort of lethargic. The train trip back to London was probably quite exhausting, though she was pleased to be home and made a tremendous fuss of Sam—who has been acting like an adolescent yobbo, attacking everyone, biting and scratching. He's no fun for Katy like this. Luckily she didn't ask about the budgie Frankie which, sadly, died.

Dr Balfour-Lynn came on Monday. He hasn't seen Katy for two weeks and was genuinely astounded by her progress. He gave her a complete examination (which she loved and during which she giggled a lot) and tested her reflexes – the hammer on her knee sent her into more fits of laughter—and she walked, turned around, sat, and stood on tip-toes for him. She can't get up off the floor by herself yet (unless she supports herself with something) but he was extremely pleased and said she is coming on magnificently. I asked about her left arm, which she still can't do much with, and he said that it might always be a little bit spastic, but I don't think so. She cares so much. I see her looking at it and analysing it, trying to work out why she does not have much control over it. She keeps her hands folded quite a lot on her lap. She wrote her name for the doctor—beautifully, I might add—but she's still not keen to write or do things of her own accord. It's her perfectionist standard, I think. She loved to do everything well before. Dr Balfour-Lynn felt it would be a help if we got some kids from school to come over each day so she has a little "gang" who will look after her when she goes back. He thought she could start school quite soon. She still asks about it six times an hour! I had been worried since she'd complained so much about headaches, but Dr Balfour-Lynn said she *will* get headaches when she's tired and was surprised she hadn't had more, considering the seriousness of her head injury.

We have started to get rid of all the paraphernalia—wheelchair, walker, hospital bed etc. Thank goodness. We have to *stop* treating her like an invalid now. We visited the hospital, as promised, and the nurses were thrilled and astonished at Katy's progress. The sister from the Children's Ward was especially delighted that she was talking so much. She said she had been convinced that Katy would not regain her talking reflex, that she would be dumb. I'm glad she didn't tell us. Katy talks more and more each day. It's still whispery but very intelligent, though she has little or no inflection. It's somewhat of a monotone.

I was away for a few days this week with *Mrs Cheyney* in Birmingham. Now I see what people mean when they say they see a difference in her after three days, even if it is minor—she is *much* more co-ordinated and is speaking more and looks even prettier and plumper than before. I had bought some new dresses for her in Brighton and she looks terribly chic with her short hair (which she hates). I took her to the hairdresser with me and asked her if she wanted her hair washed and blow-dried to make it look fuller, and she said, "Yes, Mummy, I'm fed up with looking like a punk rocker!" She enjoyed having a fuss made over her inch and a half of hair and said she liked the smell when the girl put setting lotion on to style it. Well, there isn't much hair, but what there is looks cute and she looked lovely afterwards. We have had long discussions this week about whether or not she should get her ears pierced. She wants to but is scared and asks over and over again, "Will it hurt?" When we say "No" each time she says, "When will I get my ears pierced, Mummy?" At least eight times today.

WEEK 12

We went to Jackie and Oscar's for Sunday tea. The whole family and many close friends were there. John and Jan, Claire, Nicky, and John's mother Sarah, who was moved to tears when she saw Katy and how well she was walking and how brave she is. Her eyes kept filling with tears and she'd say, "It's a miracle, a miracle—she's so beautiful!" She is a sweet lady. It was she who sent Rabbi Turetsky to see us and he who had the synagogue have special services for her. Katy ate like a horse and joined in all the fun with relish. It was Hazel's birthday and she had many presents. Katy had made her a card and enjoyed the social family scene and sang "Happy Birthday" with glee, though not too much voice.

On Monday we finally decided—after a few more thousand questions about "Will it hurt?"—that Katy should have her ears pierced. I took her to Selfridges, and first we went to the children's department where we bought a pink party dress as she was going to Jade Jagger's ninth birthday party the next day. In the toy department I said she could buy what she wanted with her accumulation of pocket money over the past eleven weeks which, at fifty pence a week, comes to £5.50. She chose something costing £28! I don't believe the price of toys, but I can't deny her anything right now. We met Jackie and Rory and Tiffany and went to the ear-piercing booth. Katy was nervous, and so was I! Tiffany went first and Katy watched intently. Then, when it was her turn, she pulled away just as the needle went through her lobe and she screamed with pain. After all she's gone through it seems weird that a teeny-weeny jab should hurt her so much. Afterwards, though, she was extremely pleased with her looks and kept asking when she could wear diamond earrings!

She has been doing all her exercises very well, but at the same time I'm aware of how much more she needs to do. When your child could run, hop, skip, jump, stand on one leg and do somersaults it's strange to have to watch her re-learn how to do them. I feel enormously sad that this terrible accident has robbed her of four or six months of her eight active years. I worry so much about the outcome. Too much, I know. As Ron says, I'm a fool to worry, and she's going to be fine, and her bravery and spirit are wonderful to watch. But she can also be a stubborn little thing, and when she's told to do something she doesn't want to, she goes on strike!

Mrs Cheyney opened in London this week. Katy looked exquisite in her new pink dress, with little gold studs in her pierced ears. She sat through the whole performance in the dress circle and then came backstage afterwards, with a big smile and folding a sweet card she had made in her own writing. Sensibly, since my dressing-room was full of flowers and well-wishers quaffing champagne, she said she was tired and went home. We had to smuggle her out through the front of the house since there were photographers backstage clamouring for a photo of her, and I do not want her exploited.

WEEK 13

I feel I have hardly seen Katy at all in the last couple of weeks, being in Birmingham and working with *Mrs Cheyney* on rehearsals and doing publicity for my beauty book. Both are going well and the London opening of *Mrs Cheyney* was very exciting—but now it's time to write some more and spend more time at home. Katy has been progressing, but of course she's still not better. I have been quite depressed about it. We were staying at the country house for a couple of days. The leaves were falling and autumn is here. Summer was spent beside her bed in a hospital in Acton, and in traffic jams between there and central London.

On Sunday we went to the opening of a small flat in the hospital. The money to build it has been raised by the hospital's League of Friends, and it can accommodate two sets of parents or relatives of people in the Intensive Care Unit. The Chairman of the League of Friends said that its completion had been inspired by the realization that great good could come from parents being able to be with their seriously injured children, as we were with Katy, and she asked Katy and me to open the flat officially. It was a very joyous occasion.

Katy is now what could be called slightly eccentric. This worries me more than it seems to worry Ron or the doctors. She asks the same questions *endlessly* and it takes enormous patience and understanding to cope. I must be a selfish pig because I'm so overwrought from the opening and the amount of work I've done with television shows, interviews, photo sessions and publicity that I crave some time to myself to sit and stare into space or just potter about. However, any spare time must go to Katy as I know how much she needs me and, of course, I need her. But oh, why do I feel this low now, when she's doing so beautifully and I have successful career things happening? Perhaps it's a reaction to everything that has happened in the past three months. I desperately want Katy to be as she was. I get a lump in my throat too often when I look at her sweet, brave face and her head with the hair all chopped off, and at her walking with her hands clasped in front of her because her left hand is still quite spastic and she is aware of it and so keeps it under control. And I compare her with how

111

she used to be—long blonde hair, jumping, active, busy. She can be all these things again and in many ways she is, but there is still so very, very far to go.

When I think of the early days of the accident I get physically sick and feel almost faint. I cannot believe we nearly lost her. I wake up in the night in a panicky nightmare thinking of those horrendous days. Ron and I must have had nerves of steel. I don't know how we coped. Seeing her now with her friend Charlotte, lying on the floor on a cushion watching children's TV in her usual position, just as she used to, I am astounded that she is here. Yet I feel so ambivalent. I'm petrified that she will stay like this even though I see she improves each week.

She never stops talking or keeps still. Her voice is good but slow and so is her vocabulary. Her posture is still a little funny. Her shoulders are hunched and she sticks out her tummy, but her co-ordination is improving rapidly. She has to be watched *all* the time, as her will to try and do everything is intense. At the same time (being a Gemini like me) she becomes impatient and aggravated when she can't do things properly. Her attention span is about one and a half seconds. We want her to do more work—writing and reading and things—but she doesn't want to do anything. I want to do everything I can to make her well but she just won't always be co-operative. Debbie is having her do all sorts of complicated exercises now in her physio sessions, but one night Katy cried and sobbed. "I don't want to do exercises any more." She doesn't want to do anything. What can we do?

I try to be positive all the time, but I am desperately worried about her. In the newspaper today I read about a woman who drove her husband and her son over a cliff because her husband had had a brain injury three months before. His personality had changed so much that it had ruined all their lives. I'm haunted by the fear that this might have happened to Katy. When she asks me the same question for the thirtieth

112

time in an hour I sometimes think she is a little crazy. But surely this is only temporary, as Mr Illingworth would not have such confidence otherwise? It is a matter of everyone around her being as sensible and down-to-earth, as helpful and placating as possible. The child has been through sheer and bloody hell, and we *have* to dredge up the incredible patience we need to help her get over it, and not let her know we expect too much. Tara is wonderful with Katy but I don't ever have any time to spend with her, and at just seventeen a girl needs her mother.

Judy Kass, Ron's sister, arrived from Los Angeles and I wanted to hear her say how fabulous Katy was, but she was non-committal and said she hadn't known what to expect but that she thought her voice was good. Everything adds to the depression. Ron is very positive all the time about Katy, but I think he knows something more than he is telling me.

WEEK 14

In the country.

Everything seems rosier when we are here. Katy loves it. She blossoms. For one thing, we can let her have much more freedom. I crave a piece of chocolate, but I have given it up until Katy is completely better. She has been adorable this week and I feel incredibly appreciative and filled with joy that she's so lovely, gentle and beautiful. She lay in bed with me one night after I had given her a bath. I had washed her hair and painted her fingernails and she cuddled her new toy lamb, obviously delighted that I didn't have to go to work that night. I noticed in the bath that her body is out of condition. There are fatty rolls around her tum and her bottom is getting plump. We must work on that with exercise. More work!

113

WEEK 15

I got sick with rage this week when I was told that there is a feeling in Fleet Street in certain quarters that I am "cashing in" on Katy's accident because of the amount of publicity it has been generating.

I am appalled and upset. Of *course* I talk about every detail of Katy's progress to anyone, including journalists—it's just about the only thing I've been thinking about for the past three and a half months—and even though I don't really want to talk to journalists about it, I am now so thrilled by her improvement that when they constantly ask me questions about her I am proud to answer. The fact is that I am more proud of what she is doing than anything *I* have ever achieved. She is the most important thing, and nothing else matters. It's sad, really. My faith in human beings had become so strong because of how wonderfully everyone supported Ron and me during those terrible days, and I find it impossible that Fleet Street tongues should wag in such an evil way—as though Katy's situation is something we should be *ashamed* of?? I immediately cancelled every interview and radio spot I was supposed to do, much to the dismay of the PR people for my beauty book, as most of the interviews had been scheduled before Katy's accident because of the book launch.

There is good news about Katy, though. Mr Illingworth came to see her. It's two weeks since he last visited and, to quote him, he was "very encouraged by her progress". I told him that since we were with her all the time we couldn't really see any change from day to day, but he said there was a definite and absolute improvement, her walking and balance were *much* better and he could see her true personality emerging more and more. He said he would put her at 85 per cent and was fairly confident that in three months she would be a hundred per cent. He still felt, though, that she might always have some little problem with the dexterity of her left hand, and he was unable to predict the outcome of her half-dilated right pupil. He warned us about her becoming too fat (her appetite is enormous) as this is common to people with her injuries. To sum up, he said that her progress was as he had expected but *much* faster! This is wonderful but I must curb my impatience. Last week when I was putting photos in the family album I got all worked up looking at the pictures of her sports day in July, when she was running and jumping and competing, looking healthily flushed and athletic.

Mr Illingworth said that if Katy hates the physio sessions so much (which she does) there was no reason to continue them as long as she had plenty of day-to-day activity like long walks and helping with housework. She was gleeful when I told her. I decided to take her with me to my exercise class next week. Her headmistress came to see her and suggested that Katy goes to the fourth-form library session to see all her school-mates. She was excited about this but kept asking, "Will I have to work?" We assured her that she would not, and she heaved a huge sigh of relief.

She and her cousins Rory and Tiffany came to the matinée of *Mrs Cheyney* with Fiona. Simon came into my dressing room at the interval for tea and Katy was very proud to show him off to the others, although she spent most of her time sticking her tongue out at him and pushing him about. Her hair is starting to look good—it just needs about another inch and it will be in the latest short style from Paris. She is extremely clothes conscious and chooses her outfits with care. One day I took her with me for a walk down Mount Street to the bank. She likes to see my safe-deposit box and look at my treasures, but I think she knows that she is the greatest treasure of all! She has started writing funny little notes to me as she used to before the accident. One morning she came in with my breakfast tray and a note which said, "Please try not to make a noise with

115

your teeth when you crunch your toast!"

Rabbi Turetsky came to the play on Thursday night and talked about what an absolute miracle her recovery is. He said that when he first saw her after three days in Intensive Care it was the saddest sight he had ever seen. He feels definitely that the faith and strength Ron and I poured into her contributed enormously to her progress. I know that is true. Although we had our moments of doubt at the time, we never allowed ourselves to believe that she would be anything but all right.

On Saturday we went to the country house. We walked up the hill and we had a long conversation. She still can't run but she was kicking her feet through the fallen autumn leaves and picking up bits of frost. Cars kept whizzing by and there was no kerb so I had to keep on lifting her up on to the grass verge. She became rather tired after half a mile and wanted me to carry her—really! It would not have been easy for she weighs seventy pounds and was wearing boots and an anorak. Luckily a friend drove by and gave us a lift back. He said if we'd walked all the way to the house I would probably have collapsed during the second show tonight. I took the 2.40 train back to London. Katy was a tiny bit sad and decided to go to bed and have a rest before Daphne Clinch arrived to have tea with her. I know Ron takes great care of her, but I called from the theatre and she was fine and very happy to see Daphne who adores her.

WEEK 16

I took Katy to school for a visit and she was absolutely lionized! All of the children gathered around her oohing and saying, "Oh Katyana, we're so happy to see you!" She clung on to me for dear life at first, and sat on my lap squashing me. I got the kids talking and they started showing me their school books (some of their handwriting was worse than Katy's is now), then I casually went over to talk to the teacher and left Katy to queen it. They were thrilled to see her and asked questions about the accident, which she answered in a practically normal voice. She is very mischievous now and seems better around other children. I think she plays up the fact that she has been seriously injured. I heard her say to one boy, "How can you expect me to do that when I've had a bad accident?" She didn't really want to go back to school, but I thought it was about time to begin the process and made arrangements for her to sit in on a class. I left her there one morning with Fiona—and Fiona called half an hour later and said Katy was putting her hand up to answer questions and joining in and writing and enjoying herself hugely! Not only that but doing excellent work! I was thrilled. She came home at lunchtime as she was tired. I looked at her work books and they were superb. Such neat work, both in English and maths, and she had been given two stars. This is a good step, but we mustn't rush her as she must regain complete confidence and not take a step back.

I took her to my exercise class and she loved it. She really had a work-out, doing bending and stretching for over an hour, and then she played catchball with the instructor, Dreas, and even tried some of the machines. Dreas said she has a lot of tension in the back of her neck which is maybe why she gets such bad headaches and why her shoulders are hunched. He gave her an after-exercise massage and her posture definitely improved. *And* her headaches seem to have stopped. She hasn't had one for nearly a week. Dreas suggested I take her to an osteopath, which I did. He was very gentle and gave her the special massage technique that he uses and said there was absolutely nothing wrong with her that would not get better. She also went to the eye specialist, who gave her eyes a complete check-up. He said she could not read the last two lines of very fine print at the bottom of the eye chart, and that her right pupil, which is still dilated, *does* react to stimulus and he feels it will eventually get better, too. Three cheers!

I had designed a green velvet dress with a white lace collar which Raymond Ray made for Katy. We were going to use a photograph of her wearing it for our Christmas card—we would obviously have to send hundreds as I wanted to thank personally all the people who sent us letters and comforted us. On Tuesday I took Katy to Selfridges where she was photographed in front of two Christmas trees, and she looked stunning. It was 5.30 so the place was deserted except for window-dressers. She trotted around looking at Snow White and the Seven Dwarfs in the Grotto with great interest, remembering the movie she saw a month ago. Then she met Father Christmas—the most wonderful Santa Claus I've ever seen, with a big red nose and a wheezy voice. He must have been an actor because he said to me, "Hello, Mrs Cheyney." He was delightful with Katy. She sat at his feet, looked up at him with trust and whispered to him that what she really wanted for Christmas was a pony! Dear God, that's all we need now! I think her getting involved in riding again, particularly jumping, would cause me to have a nervous breakdown—which I sometimes feel I am veering towards in any case.

We tried to think of what to put into our Christmas card and came up with:

OUR DREAMS CAME TRUE THIS CHRISTMAS
WE HOPE YOURS WILL TOO

One night a young Australian doctor from the Central Middlesex Hospital came backstage with his wife. He told me that all of the staff—doctors, nurses etc.—at the hospital were impressed and amazed by what Ron and I did when Katy was in there. He said that many of them truly believed that she would not ever come out of the coma and, if she did, they were positive she would be seriously disabled, a vegetable, or maybe blind or deaf or mute. I got the shudders. His wife said that each day he would come home with reports of what we were doing, and was astonished by our optimism. Well, it proves that optimism and faith *do* work.

ONWARD!

It's Sunday and we are now in the country. It's cold, wet and windy, but Katy is so cheery and improving that it's wonderful just to sit and watch her. At the moment she is wearing a pale lilac jump-suit that we bought her in Paris in August (oh dear!) and a white shirt with a dark lilac bow that Fiona has tied at the neck like a little bow-tie. Her hair is growing well and her fringe almost reaches her eyebrows. It's much darker than it was before, but it is quite well shaped and sets off her gold earrings. Her right pupil is only about fifty per cent dilated now, and often it is hardly noticeable. She is sitting at her old school desk in her bedroom absorbed in writing a letter to her friends Victoria and Samantha in Los Angeles. It is an excellent letter, very good neat writing, well constructed, with only a few tiny mistakes. It says, "I know my writing is a bit shaky but I am feeling fine, I hope you are too." When she is encouraged to do things like write and draw, she does them very well. Her intelligence seems to have increased and her sense of humour and perception are acute. She said to me the other day when I had on some pearls, "Are those Mrs Ebley's pearls?" (Mrs Ebley is a character in *Mrs Cheyney*) and when I told her they were mine she said that they didn't seem to be my style—and anyway she didn't know I owned any!

At the theatre last night I found out that because the business for *Mrs Cheyney* is not too good the show will probably be closing soon. Therefore, because Ron and I are investors, the producers are setting my weekly salary against our investment losses. This means I am doing eight performances a week from now until we close for no money *at all*. I was so upset that instead of acting I *really* cried on stage when Simon pretended to slap me! It is almost too much to cope with on top of everything else. Our expenses for all the things we need for Katy are so high we really need that money. And, of course, I have to continue performing, which is humiliating.

I took her for a walk in the country today in the pouring rain, and she walked very fast and climbed on to the grass verges and jumped. But she *won't* run. I wonder why? Sometimes I just stare at her in wonder. It seems like such a miracle. I realize more and more all the time how terribly serious and potentially fatal it almost was. It seems strange that I couldn't think of that then and could only think positively. Perhaps I knew subconsciously how ghastly it was but wouldn't admit it. I still wake up two or three times a week with a nightmare feeling recalling those early days and weeks. Usually I take a Valium and manage to go back to sleep. I feel *terribly* tired and exhausted, but the show must go on.

WEEK 17

On Sunday I felt totally drained after two performances on Saturday, but dragged myself out to have lunch with friends at our local pub. My sinus condition had been getting worse and it suddenly flared up. My eye started to water, I had a searing pain in my head and had to leave in the middle of lunch. I didn't feel any better at home, so lay down and took all sorts of potions.

The week has basically been good for Katy mentally, but not so good physically—mostly because she developed a slight cold and has had to take lots of medication—but her humorous side is coming out more and more, and Ron believes she is actually more intelligent than before the accident. Certainly the writing in the composition she wrote at school on Tuesday is much clearer, neater and has more strength and depth to it than the one she wrote in July—although there are a few more spelling mistakes. Her teacher gave her another star and Fiona said she did very well, though she did not wish to do French and wanted Fiona to stay with her all the time.

On Saturday, we took her to the races at Sandown Park where I was presenting a trophy to the winner of the 2.30 race and having lunch with various VIPs. Katy sat at a different table with Ron and behaved extremely well, in spite of lots of people crowding around her and fussing about. She said to the girl she was sitting next to, "Look at my hand shaking—I look like an old lady!" This was because of the cough medicine she had been taking. It's debilitating. She made three bets and won two of them, clearing £11. She was exceedingly thrilled! Then we were ushered into the Royal Box to meet the Queen Mother, who was most charming and Katy was delighted to meet her. She whispered to me, did I think the Queen Mother had heard about her accident? I didn't know, but then I heard one of the Ladies-in-Waiting asking about Katy at length and she seemed to know about the accident.

After the next race, the Clerk of the Course asked Katy and me to follow the Queen Mother and himself and go to the winners' enclosure where the QM was to present the trophy. We took a short cut through the kitchen and then walked across the back part of the track, thus losing Ron who missed a great photograph of Katy and the Queen Mother!

When I look at Katy now, lying on her tummy at the bottom of my bed, her chin in her hands, I see the *exact* same little girl who was doing *exactly* the same thing on 29th July, three days before the accident. Her face, expression, weight and personality all seem identical. Of course there is still quite a bit of physical disability but it's clearly coming along in a slow but sure way. The Polaroids are the most emphatic proof. I take them constantly and am always comparing them to the ones of a week or a month previously. They are an excellent guide to her progress.

WEEK 18

On Sunday, Tessa Kennedy had a particularly special Thanksgiving Mass for Katy at her church in Windsor. Father Fontenari, the Italian priest, talked to the congregation about the little girl they had all prayed for during the past four months, saying that she was so much better today and that Jesus had saved her. Then he asked Katy to come up to the altar to receive his blessing. She was very sweet and did it immediately. She was a bit shy, but Milica took her hand and they both stood there in front of the congregation while I watched with such pride and with *such* a lump in my throat. It was all I could do to stop sobbing out loud. Tessa was also very moved and so was Ron. As a staunch Catholic, Tessa has *still* not had a drink since Katy's accident—that is what she chose to give up. I have not eaten one bit of chocolate, but it is not such a sacrifice as booze! These pledges stand until Katy's complete recovery.

Jean and Robin Illingworth came to Thanksgiving Lunch afterwards at Tessa and Elliott's. Mr Illingworth brought Katy a present, a hand puppet of a monkey which she immediately christened Bananas. He said it was for her to use to work her left hand. He was most happy to see her, although he felt that her physical co-ordination and walking were not as good as two weeks ago, and he thought this was due to the antihistamine cough medicine she has been taking because of her cold. She is very susceptible to drugs. He said not to worry. She was doing excellently, more or less as he predicted. He felt that the major part of the improvement would take place over the next two months and the other residual things (dilated right pupil, shaky left hand and balance problem) would take a year or so. A year—what an eternity! Still, since Katy is now ninety per cent fit and almost died four months ago, I suppose we should consider ourselves lucky.

Mr Illingworth feels that Katy *must* start school properly, and she has agreed to go on 11th January when the spring term starts. I hope we will not have too many problems then, although I do anticipate a few. I've told her she needn't do sports or dancing or handiwork until she feels up to it.

Mr Illingworth told Ron we were fortunate that a brilliant young registrar (who worked under Mr Illingworth and Mr Rice Edwards) took the call from Heatherwood Hospital and it was decided it would be best to transfer Katy to the Central Middlesex where they specialized in her kind of injury. This is the first event that contributed to saving her life.

WEEK 19

Sunday was a red-letter day—Katy ran! I had been urging her to run for several weeks but each time she refused, said she didn't know how to, couldn't remember how to. She had her new Kickers on, and when we went out for our Sunday walk I said, "Come on, Katy, I'm sure you can run in those!"—and off she went, with me holding her hand, down the lane. It was actually more of a kind of half gallop-cum-trot-cum-skip than proper running, but I was excited—and quite out of breath as she went faster than me. We ran several times, each time with her holding on tightly to my hand with her left one. Then she got adventurous and while I was picking holly she ran by herself. The progress seems terribly slow these days, but people who haven't seen her for a week or two see a big difference.

John Lennon was murdered this week. His death brought back to me with frightening clarity just how ephemeral all our lives are and how a matter of a millimetre, whether a knock on the head or a bullet wound, can mean the difference between life and death.

WEEK 20

This week began horrifically. On Monday, Ron woke me up by asking the name of Simon Williams' daughter. "It's Amy," I said sleepily. "Oh good. I'm so glad—I thought it was Flora," he said. "Flora's Lucy's daughter," I said, rapidly awakening. Ron, grim-faced, showed me the *Daily Mail*. "CHILD AND FATHER FEARED DROWNED IN THAMES . . . the eight-year-old daughter of actress etc. etc. . . ." I couldn't believe it was true. I called Rod Tyler, who confirmed that Flora and her father had been drowned on Sunday night while Simon and Lucy were doing *Night of a Hundred Stars* just down the road at the National Theatre. Simon's words came back to me, all the many times he came to visit Katy in hospital, bringing his and Lucy's children. "Do you know, Katy, you ruined Lucy's and my holiday in Portugal with the children? When we heard that you were ill we used to sit on the beach and watch our kids playing in the waves and get very, very nervous that they might drown. We didn't take our eyes off them because of what happened to you."

Simon, who loves children so much, who was so helpful and supportive when Katy was ill, had lost Flora who was almost like one of his own children. I kept thinking of the two of them, Katy and Flora, in Chichester this summer, rushing backstage and visiting us all in our dressing rooms, playing little tricks on us and giggling. I spent most of the day hugging Katy and looking at her, thinking of our luck and how it could so easily have been different. I had been beginning to get despondent about how long it all seems to be taking and now—God—I felt lucky to have her at all. I didn't leave her side all day. Felt enormous sadness for Simon and Lucy.

Spoke to him. He said Lucy was being magnificent. For three days Alistair Cameron played Simon's role, and the whole cast was depressed, thinking of Simon and Lucy all the time.

It has been a good week for Katy, though. She went to school twice, once for a morning of lessons and once for the end-of-term party. At first she didn't want to go to it, but Fiona stayed with her and she had lots of fun. Her headmistress seems to think that she has become a more outgoing child since the accident and is very pleased that she will be back next term. It seems strange that the accident should have helped her personality and made her more sure of herself, more confident and funnier. She is also much more affectionate than she was before, and now her normal temper is also starting to emerge. Thank God—I don't want her to be a Pollyanna for ever! When two of us were both calling out for her, she appeared outraged in the door of her bathroom shouting, "I'm in the loo—can't a person go to the loo in peace without everyone yelling and disturbing her?" Then she went back in with a cross face. Ron said she sounds just like me!

I took her to the hairdresser's again, and they all saw an improvement in her. She is quite cheeky now and chatted away to YoYo, who does her hair, like a sophisticated thirty-five-year-old. On Thursday she stayed for tea, supper and overnight with Rory at my sister's house. I was nervous as it was her first time away for the night, but Jackie said she was wonderful. On Friday we went back to the hospital where we presented three thousand pounds-worth of life-support machines to the Premature Baby Unit on behalf of the charity BLISS. Dozens of Fleet Street's finest were there and were allowed in three at a time to photograph Katy and me and a little premature baby. I was amazed that so many members of the press showed up and printed Katy's story yet *again*. When some of the journalists asked me why I was there I told them that I felt a debt of gratitude to the hospital that I could never repay. *That* is for sure. They virtually saved Katy's life and nothing I could ever do for them could compensate for saving her. I became moved and quite upset. It brought it all back to me again. I took Katy to the Children's Ward where we saw the sister, and Pat and Breda and many of the other nurses who clamoured around and said how wonderful she was. I think she is secretly rather pleased with all the attention, but it makes her shy too and she buries her face in my shoulder.

Ron has gone to a health farm for six days to lose weight (he's gained forty pounds since the accident). I wish I could have even one day of rest. I am desperately tired. Doing the show eight times a week, and Christmas shopping, and watching over Katy is draining me. Plus business is bad and it's debilitating and humiliating performing for no salary. The cast are aware, and are sympathetic. I still have awful sinus trouble, and toothache, and now my eyes have gone red and bloodshot and my eyelids are sore and swollen. My voice went totally on Friday night. It was quite a scary experience being on stage and just a croak coming out. The doctor said my vocal cords had packed up from sheer exhaustion, overwork and stress, and that I must slow down. Great. Easier said than done. I mean, apart from everything else, Christmas is coming. I'm feeling sorry for myself again. Shape up, Joan!

Dear Joan and Ron,
Thanks ever so much for the cards. Sorry you had to wait for a reply but I thought I had sent it till I came across the letter this morning.

We were really thrilled to bits about Katy. She looks so well, fit and healthy that it makes you marvel at the human body. There's a little girl in the same condition as our two girls were, Joan, and when we went to the hospital for our Tracy's check up the nurses told me about her. She lives in Durham and it was only half an hour's drive away so we went to see her.

It was quite awful to see and brought back all we felt at the time but the mother was over the moon to see our Tracy as she knew all about her from the nurses and she said she felt a lot better as you know yourself what dreadful thoughts you have at a time like that. Anyway to get back to the point of telling all this I took the photos of our Tracy but also the ones of Katy so you can tell Katy she has helped someone the same as herself.

When we went for her check up she was discharged—no more medication and she does not need even to be in contact with the hospital ever again and it's only nine months now she is completely back to normal apart from a slight shakiness in her left hand of a morning and which the doctor has said will go with time. It seems such a long time ago and so unreal now.

I'll close now, give Katy a big kiss from us and tell her our Tracy has the card she sent on her bedroom wall.

I hope Katy likes her book. Our Tracy likes this one and we wanted to get her a little something to keep and read and as a memento it was quite a struggle as I'm sure Katy has everything you could think of. We are also thrilled to bits that things turned out for you the way they did and the hard work you and Ron put in paid off.

Love,
Dot and Alan

Dear Katy

I thank you for your letter I got it on Thursday.

I too like the frill on the top of your dress.

I do like your Snoopy paper. I hope you like this muppet show paper I chose this myself too. My mum has just been doing my hair do you like your hair short? I don't. Are you going to let yours grow long. I will close now.

Lots of love
Tracy

These letters are heartwarming.

127

WEEKS 21 and 22

Sunday, 28th December: I am vastly depressed and frightened. We took Katy out to dinner last night at Mr Kai's with Milica, Tessa, Elliott, Father Rooney and others. She was fabulous— funny, full of life, gregarious and talkative. We arrived in the country at two in the morning and she complained of a piercing headache. I gave her Veganin and she got into bed with me. She woke at eight with another ghastly headache. Another Veganin and back to sleep until eleven. All day she has been unwell and in agony on and off with her headache. I felt weak, unable to cope—and frightened. *Why* does she keep getting these horrible pains in her head? Maybe because she was over-excited by Christmas. Or is there something more seriously wrong with her? Like permanent brain damage . . . I can't bear to think about it and push it to the back of my mind.

She was wonderful over Christmas, which was eventful to say the least. On Christmas Eve we wrapped presents and put them under the tree, and then Katy helped me set the table for the buffet supper. Rod and Maggie, Eve, Leslie and Adam Bricusse came, and Tara and Sacha were there. Katy stayed up late and had a super time. In the morning there was much excitement with lots of presents. She certainly did well in *that* department. Understandably. Then on to Jackie's for another huge family get-together, lunch and another hundred or so presents. On Boxing Day she went to a pantomime—*Aladdin*—with Ron, Tiffany and Rory, then stayed overnight at Jackie's.

So she is probably having a reaction to all that. I had to stroke her head to get her to sleep tonight. Just as I thought I'd got her off and was creeping out of the room, she would awake and complain of more pain. Finally I brought her into my bed and she cheered up while we watched Celia Johnson and Trevor Howard in a play on television. After a while she

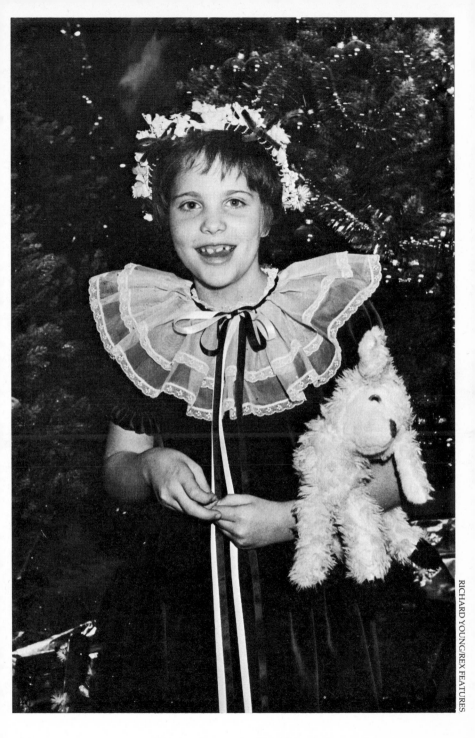

"Our dreams came true this Christmas.
We hope yours will too."

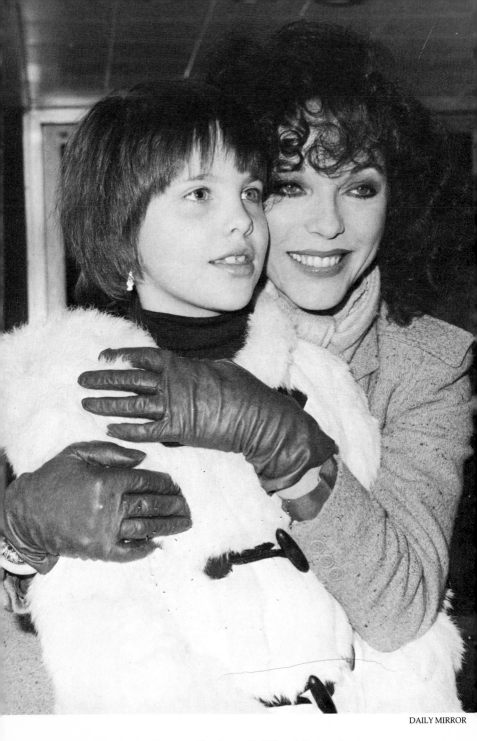

FIVE MONTHS: Our beautiful Katy is beginning to
emerge again.

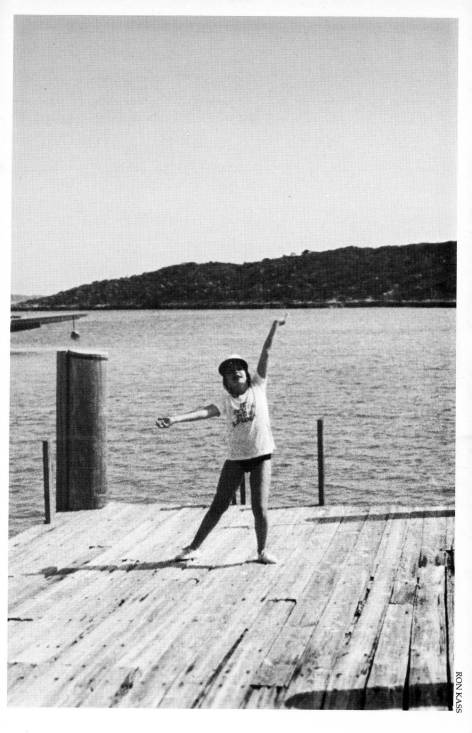

SIX MONTHS: Katy starts to show her old vigorous personality
on holiday in the Bahamas.

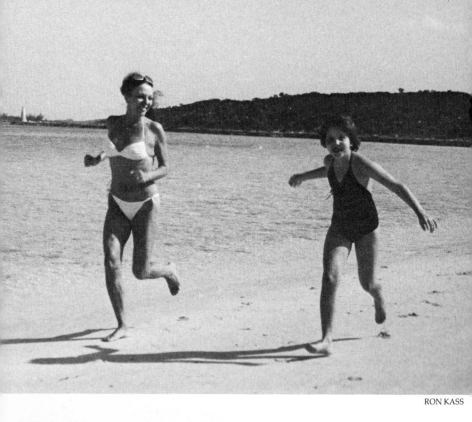

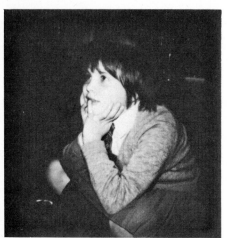

Above: She runs properly for
the first time.
Left: Back at school.

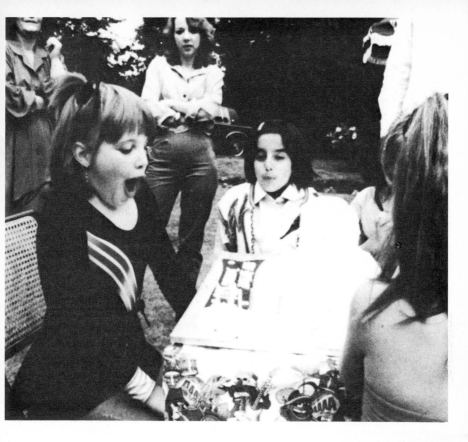

TEN MONTHS: Happy Ninth Birthday! 20 June 1981.

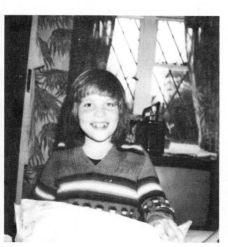

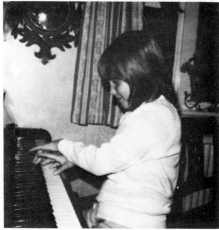

Onward!

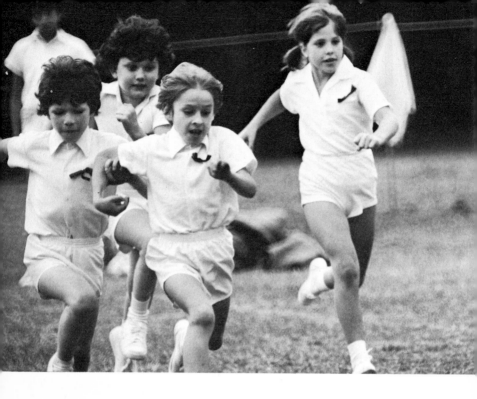

ELEVEN MONTHS: Katy's school sports day.

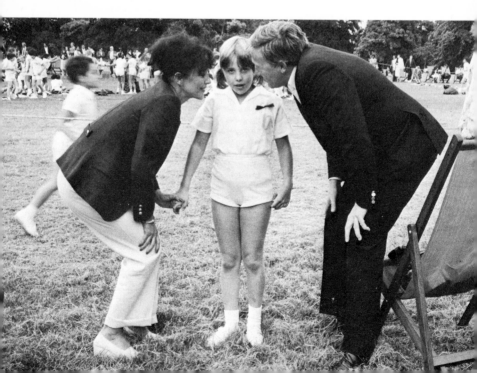

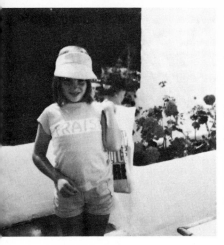

ONE YEAR

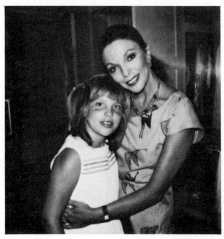

The day Katy passed the entrance examination for her new American school – with 78%!

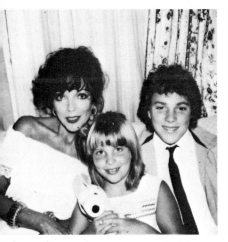

THIRTEEN MONTHS: with Sacha.

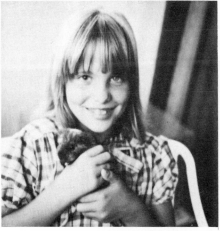

FOURTEEN MONTHS

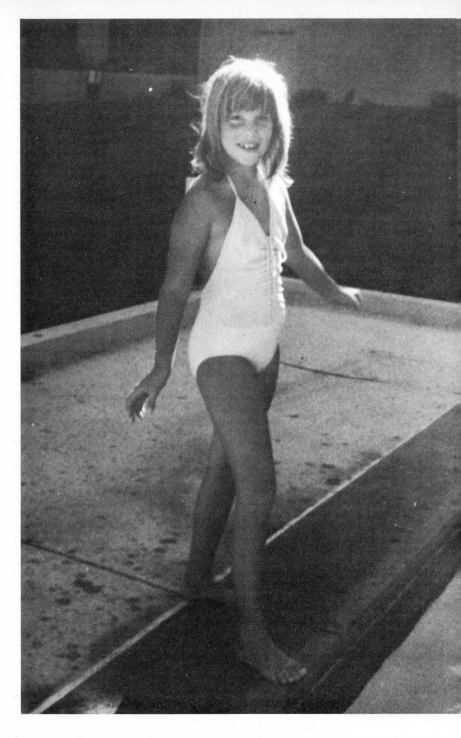

FIFTEEN MONTHS: Katyana Kennedy Kass.
"She has come a long, long way."

said, "These old English people are so typical, aren't they?" "Typical of what?" I asked. "Just typical," she said observantly. Then a fat Indian lady came on screen and Katy said, "She's probably so enormous because she eats roasted alligators and fried hedgehogs and boiled cats." Quite an inventive remark about an Indian menu for an eight-year-old child!

New Year's Day 1981: On Tuesday we went to John Lewis to buy Katy's new school uniform. It's thrilling to think she is going to be starting school in two weeks. She is really looking forward to it and looked gorgeous with pink flushed cheeks and a mischievous twinkle in her eyes. Even her walking seemed to be better—in the shoe department she walked around in new shoes and the walk was practically perfect. It was wonderful to do something as ordinary as buying a school uniform. Several people came up for autographs and asked her how she was feeling. Again she wondered why she was so famous, why everyone knew who she was, and was it because mummy was famous or because she was famous? She rather likes all the attention, but is *not* spoiled by it.

New Year's Eve, Ron and I took her to Mr Kai's with Tara and a group of friends. We sang "Auld Lang Syne" and I prayed that 1981 would be better for us all than 1980. Katy drank half a glass of champagne and got very giggly.

It is five months since the accident, and I would say she is about ninety per cent normal. My fears that she will never be completely normal again still crop up. She has two or three good days and then a day of headaches, listlessness and just mooning around and looking bored. I feel very thankful but very depressed too. All the experts say that the last ten per cent will be the hardest hurdle to overcome.

Katy

THE SIXTH MONTH: *January 1981*

It is over five and a half months since the accident. Katy is eating a tangerine, delicately pulling the white fibre off each section while watching some handicapped people on television. It is the Year of the Disabled. A severely spastic boy is in a new special chair donated by the *Blue Peter* programme. He is about fourteen years old. Katy is exceedingly interested—as am I, for she could so easily have been as badly disabled, if not more so, than this boy. How very fortunate she is, lying there at the bottom of my bed, looking around, opening a box of sweets, scribbling in a notepad, eating a tangerine. She is still a little shaky when she moves, her speech is still somewhat slow and monotonous, and her laughter sometimes sounds crazy, but I suddenly see another breakthrough from three or four weeks ago. This boy on the television is so brave and so delighted with his new chair, which will enable him to do all sorts of things he couldn't do before. He is determined to get a hundred per cent out of the sixty per cent chance he has. I think he is wonderful, but—although I know it sounds selfish—I can't help making comparisons between him and Katy, and thanking God she won't be like him.

She started school a week ago. We were quite nervous about it. Would the other kids accept Katy as she is now? Would they make fun of her? Would she be able to cope with all the stairs and the other kids jostling her? Would the teachers be understanding and not press her too much? She's a perfectionist and it was so important to build up her confidence and not criticize her or let her think her work was below par. She was extremely confident, more than before, but she had some trepidation about school, and I didn't blame her.

This television programme shows how much disabled people accept their handicaps and can be treated just like anyone else, and I know that is true of Katy, even though her handicap is temporary. Our concern is that she should be in no way blighted permanently as far as her mental health is concerned. She is sensitive and acutely perceptive and we don't want her to get hurt. I had a long talk with her headmistress before she started school and she was very aware of the situation and had interesting ideas about how to handle it. She said that this term she and the other teachers would not expect anything scholastically and would not push her in any way. Now, after five school days, Katy seems to be loving it. Not one headache since the New Year and she is walking and running much straighter. She does her homework carefully each night and her stories, essays, drawings and spelling are excellent. Maths is not so good—but she was never good at it before.

Mrs Cheyney is closing soon, which is sad but at the same time I am desperately in need of a rest, and I've been performing without salary for over a month. I have not been sleeping well and woke up today feeling ghastly. Dr Eppel came and said I am an emotional and physical wreck. The strain of Katy's illness, plus the play and all the other pressures have finally got me down. He gave me medication and said I couldn't perform tonight and maybe not tomorrow either. He looked at Katy and was very pleased. It's been a month since he saw her.

"Do you see a change?" I asked anxiously.

"Yes, of course, and the improvement can still go on for eighteen months or so."

He made Katy stand with her hands at her sides and her eyes closed. She didn't sway at all. He said this means her balance is definitely getting better. And the pupil of her right eye is reacting more to stimuli.

Ten days later: Katy stayed overnight with Milica, whose birthday it was. She had a "pyjama party". Fiona stayed with Katy and said she enjoyed herself although some of the girls were a bit boisterous. Then Fiona said, "Two of the children asked me what was wrong with Katy." This made me really worried and I called Mr Illingworth, who came over to see her. I told him my worst fears. That, although her improvement had been so great, I could see that she still (1) had pedantic and monotonously slow speech; (2) walked and ran in a less than totally co-ordinated way; (3) had a shaky left hand which she managed to control quite well, unless she was very tired; (4) often broke out in a loud and rather crazy laugh; (5) didn't seem to have complete control over her tongue, which showed a lot of the time between her teeth.

He examined her and gave her an orange, which I peeled and she dissected delicately. He said he had been expecting that we would phone around this six-month period. He said he felt she had made the major part of her progress now and that what she is left with is what she is left with. My heart sank, and I felt more depressed than since the first days after the accident. He told us how lucky we are to have her at all. She is a miracle, and we are terribly lucky that there appears to be no mental damage at all. He explained that it is infinitely preferable to have these little minor things which she will learn to live with and adapt to, and, in time, cover up. Ron also was very reassuring and said we must realize what she has achieved, but after Mr Illingworth left I became really depressed and upset, probably exaggerated by the fact that it was the *last* of *The Last of Mrs Cheyney* that night.

I took Katy to the theatre where she helped me take down dozens of telegrams and decorations, and we played some tricks on Simon. Katy put a toy rabbit in the stage bed for him to find. All the cast were in floods of emotional tears at the end of the last show.

I talked to Ron and to Pete Cameron at length about Katy. Ron felt that Mr Illingworth was being over-cautious in saying that this was more or less as far as she would progress. Pete said he had spoken many times to a young doctor in Connecticut who specializes in dealing with comatose patients after their major recovery. He thought Katy was amazing mentally and that she was still, as he always predicted for her since before her birth, "a blessed child". Ron felt that she would recover totally, but that perhaps now she needed some special therapy to stimulate the parts of her brain which were functioning to replace the destroyed parts.

I became extremely weepy and emotional after the last night of *Mrs Cheyney*. It was like the end of a chapter—but the happy ending was not there yet. My exhaustion and general physical debilitation were not contributing to the optimism, hope and faith which I still needed. Ron says she *will* get completely better. She will—*she must*.

I went to a health farm, Stobo Castle in Edinburgh, for a few days to regenerate and rest. On the day I left I took Katy to school. She was sad I was going, and so was I. It was only for a few days but I thought I could help her more if I was strong again. At that moment I was a total physical and mental wreck with nothing to give to anyone.

On the train journey to Scotland I read a book called *Living After a Stroke* about a woman, Diana Law, who at the age of forty-odd suffered a severe stroke which, as well as many other disabilities, caused her total loss of speech. The book is most encouraging because she says that in her fight to get speech therapy clinics established, she realized that the medical profession are greatly ignorant about the incredible results that can come from therapy. To quote from her book:

> There is far too little appreciation in the medical profession of what rehabilitation can do. In only three London hospitals is there any instruction on the benefits of occupational therapy, physiotherapy and speech therapy. There is colossal medical ignorance in these areas.

Diana Law knew from her own experience that those whose speech was damaged or absent (due to strokes, head injuries, etc.) would not recover their speech in time alone. Professional help is needed to help patients, but in most cases this skilled help is not available. The medical hierarchy must become more educated about speech therapy programmes. I intend to find the best speech therapist I can to work on Katy's speech. I *know* it can be perfect again, in spite of what the doctors say.

I came back from Scotland feeling a hundred per cent better. I had talked to Katy several times by phone, and she sounded wonderful with hardly any trace of speech problems. I had a long session with an extraordinary woman called Bessie McClean who is a psychic. Ron told me about her. He saw her too and said she was uncanny in what she foretold. She concentrated for a long while as I showed her the Polaroids I keep of Katy's progress, from the first one I dared to take ten days after the accident to one of the most recent taken at Christmas with Tara and Sacha. Bessie repeated over and over: "You have *nothing* to worry about with Katy—she is going to be all right." She said she is a "special child" and Ron and I *must* keep the faith and never stop believing in God and the power of faith and prayer. She asked if the month of June had any significance and I told her Katy's birthday was in June. She foresaw a rosebud being presented and it opened into a full-blown rose. She felt this could be when Katy is completely herself again. Dare I hope?

I had been away from Katy for four days. Nothing much seems to have changed. Sometimes she seems okay and perfectly normal, but often she gets terribly impatient and irritable with those around her, particularly when she is doing her homework. Fiona says that she seems not to be able to do it by herself and needs help all the time. Ron, however, says that her grasp of things and her concept of logic are perfect, and it is just a matter of time. "You must learn to eat time," is a line from a movie I was once in called *Sea Wife*.

It is the end of the sixth month and I feel depressed. I can't wait to take Katy to the Bahamas. I took her to Marks and Spencer's yesterday to buy summer gear. She knew exactly what she wanted and was very bossy. Would not accept a flowered bikini, insisted on a chic navy-blue one-piece—rather like my Norma Kamali ones—then she dragged me round getting colour-co-ordinated T-shirts and socks. She said her colour scheme for the holiday would be navy and pink! Two assistants said how nice it was to see her up and around. She's quite famous, and it amuses her.

THE SEVENTH AND EIGHTH MONTHS: *February–March 1981*

We decided to take Katy out of school for a while as we felt that she needed some sun to get rid of her pallor and to brighten her up. She has been through so much, and swimming and running on the beach in the Bahamas would do her the world of good. There was the usual bunch of photographers at the airport. Katy handled it very well, although I feel that they become too demanding with her by insisting on photographing her dozens of times. She's a pro though, and posed uncomplainingly.

After a long flight to Miami, we had to find "the Goose" (a seven-passenger sea-plane belonging to our host, Peter de Savary) at the nearby airport. It was almost dark when we arrived at Nassau and Katy was starting to get slightly cranky and plane-sick as it was, I'll admit, quite bumpy. She went uncomplainingly to bed as soon as we got to Peter's house and went off to sleep quietly and sweetly.

During the next few days we prayed for sun but unfortunately we rarely saw it as Nassau was covered in clouds and was very windy and cold. I was so cross! Lana, Peter's girl-friend, would come outside for a few minutes at a time, shiver and go back in because it was such nasty weather. We managed to get Katy swimming again though. I had to stand in the shallow end, covered in goose bumps, encouraging her. The first day she didn't swim too well, but by the third she was doing widths and diving for coins and retrieving them all. When we first started running down the beach she did her usual sort of galloping trot, but after about an hour of this she suddenly got the gist of it again and ran—for the first time in nearly seven months my darling little girl ran! Her short hair blew in the breeze and her smile was happy and warm. She knew how good it was, for both her and us. As we walked around the streets and hotels with her, no one could see that there was anything wrong with her really. Her posture was still a bit slumped and her tongue still stuck out a bit when she talked, but it was gradually improving.

On our fourth day in Nassau her leg became very swollen from a mosquito bite. It was huge, and very painful. The doctor said that often when people have been very seriously ill their resistance is so low that the slightest thing affects them badly and they pick up any infections that are going. He said we must build her up nutritionally now and also give her lots of vitamin C and put zinc ointment on her for protection. At the end of our stay in Nassau we *finally* got some gorgeous weather. We went in Peter's plane to a tiny island, which was terribly primitive but so attractive. We lived in huts for two days! It was romantic and Katy loved it. We took rides in speedboats, picnicked and explored rocks. It was wonderful for Katy, and after spending hours a day slathering Copper-tone and sun protection creams all over her she finally got a tan and looked amazing—almost like the old Katy.

We travelled on to Los Angeles where it poured with rain for practically the whole two weeks we were there. I was miserable because the whole point of taking her out of school was to get lots of swimming *every* day, and plenty of sun and exercise. Katy spent a lot of time with her grandparents, who thought she was great, though her grandmother said she was "too plump" in the tummy and legs. Well she is, I know, but I explained that it's part of the after-effects of the injury and also because she hasn't exercised enough. She has not yet done gym or sports at school. Judy Bryer thought she looked wonderful, and Victoria (her daughter, who is the same age as Katy and my goddaughter) and Katy became even firmer friends than before. Katy stayed there overnight several times.

Then Ron and I took Katy to the Philadelphia Institute for the Achievement of Human Potential and met Dr LeWin, the founder and innovator of the clinic that specializes in the re-covery of brain-injured children, and particularly in methods of coma arousal. He initiated the CAT method of arousing patients. There is a two-year waiting list to get into the Institute for the week-long course, but we were lucky to get an hour-and-a-half meeting with the doctor, with whom we had been in contact during the time Katy had been in hospital.

He said Katy was doing "just fine" under the circumstances and much of this had to do with the extensive input Ron and I had given her in the hospital, but he said we must do *much* more for her to be as she was before. Her speech is too slow and pedantic and hasn't much inflection. He said we can improve this by making her work at it: reading out loud, shouting and practising movements with her tongue—have her eat different textures of food and savouring them. We must work on the pupil of her right eye every day with a flashlight to make it contract for one minute, and do this every three or four hours. We had worked on her eyes like this when she was in the coma, and will have to start doing it again. He said, "If that pupil isn't much better in a month, call me and I'll come and fix it for you." He said that the reason no tears appear from the tear ducts when she cries is that she is still in a sort of infant stage (babies have no tears), and although she is mentally much more advanced than an infant she has become lazy and must be *pushed* and *pushed*. Oh dear, this all sounds rather daunting.

I thought Ron and I were doing as much as we could but obviously there are miles further to go. Dr LeWin said that we *must* make her run every day, as this expands the lungs and through that her voice projection will improve. He said to *stop* doing things for her. She mustn't get into the pattern of being lazy and letting others do the things she is capable of doing herself. Dressing, washing, helping at table, dancing, games, reading out loud—all these she must now be encouraged to do. The potential is there. The mind is there. It is the physical disabilities now, however minor, that are keeping her from being a hundred per cent. And for this it is *us* who must work *her*. He put us down on his waiting list and said that if in two years there is any residual damage we must bring her back to the Institute and be prepared to work harder than we have ever done in our lives before.

Two years! God, what an eternity! I keep getting disheartened when I think of the amount of time that has gone by. Nearly seven months. It's flown, but it's been desperately hard work for all of us. I really expect and *will* her to be recovered totally within the year, which gives us about five months. I know I shouldn't set deadlines but she doesn't deserve to miss her childhood like this. From now on I shall work on her to my utmost capacity.

By the time we came back to London I noticed the following big improvements:

1. Her shoulder posture is back to normal. She keeps her shoulders straight without being told to.

2. Her tongue seems to have found its right place and doesn't peep out any more.

Dr Eppel came to visit and noticed the vast change in her from the Bahamian trip. He feels she should spend as much time in the sun as possible and do a lot of swimming and exercise. He thinks we should go home to California when winter comes as Katy will thrive more there.

THE NINTH MONTH: *April 1981*

In the country house
We have been practising what Dr LeWin preaches, and I think it's working. I definitely see a more vital and aware Katy, even in the past few days. I've been doing the eye exercise with the flashlight, and making her sing "Do re mi" from *The Sound of Music* and other songs—like nursery rhymes—and I make her project her voice. She is perfectly able to speak as fast as she did before when I *push* her, but won't in ordinary conversation. Her projection and pace, though, are practically back to normal. The left hand is still a big problem and also the balance, but I watched her run around the garden today several times and it's really quite amazing. Except that she keeps her hands out from the side of her body a bit for balance she looks almost normal. We have talked her out of a career as a show-jumper. She has now decided to be an actress! This is good because I can work with her more on her voice and movements as practice for her future career!

Ron bought her a bike but obviously it had to have stabilizers set on to it. We went for a bike ride down the lanes. She did well—but *I* nearly fell off! I also started her walking and balancing on a little ledge, while I held her hand. If I make her do something and she says, "I can't," I say, "There's no such word as Can't." And she says, "Yes there is, it's a contraction!" Who was it who said, "If you think you *can* or you *can't*

139

you're probably right"? Well we *can* and *will* make this kid perfect again. I have blanked out so much of the past seven months I'm glad I wrote it down. I remember it more like a horror story, the further away from it we get.

One week later: Katy seems to have taken several steps backwards. It's incredibly frightening and depressing. This last week she went back to the school for the new term. She must have been badly jet-lagged from the flight back from the US because by Thursday she was irritable, highly-strung, bad-tempered and sulky to both Fiona and me. On Thursday when we put on her new Brownie uniform so she could go to a Brownie meeting for the first time, we discovered that it was ten inches too long and we couldn't find her yellow tie with the Brownie badge on it. She went into a complete tantrum— yelling, flailing her arms, all the old bad signs, with her left arm going up in a funny way. She told us she hated us both and tried to cry. But still no tears come out. We tried to persuade her to wear her shorter old uniform but she refused. It was extremely upsetting, particularly since nothing seemed to comfort her. She came and lay on my bed and sulked. When I turned on the TV she snarled at the top of her voice, "Turn that thing off." It didn't make things any easier that I had to get dressed up and leave her to go to a charity occasion in aid of the Great Ormond Street Children's Hospital.

When Ron and I came home at nine she was lying in bed and seemed better. Then this morning (Friday) she came into my room before school again crying (without tears) because she hadn't learned her spelling test. We comforted her as well as we could but she was upset. When she is upset her balance goes and she seems as she was weeks ago. When she came back from school this afternoon she yelled at me, "Why didn't you pick me up from school? You promised! You must never break your promises," and stormed upstairs. I felt horribly guilty, as I do usually do what I promise. I calmed her down but her fuse was *very* short. We went to pick up Ron at his office, then we drove down to the country house which she loves. But once there she was tired, grumpy, snappy, un-co-ordinated, her left arm going right up almost into a hook over her shoulder. I was in despair. We played dominoes and she got fed up very quickly, then a card game and she got bored and restless. We cuddled on the sofa and I stroked her like a cat, which she usually loves. During dinner she looked tired and cross and I put her to bed.

Ron and I both felt horribly depressed and upset. We discussed that it was probably (hopefully) extreme exhaustion as we have only been back from the States for nine days, and she's had full days at school. Also, now that Ron is working again he comes home later and Katy doesn't see him as much. And we went out to dinner parties four nights in a row, so maybe that upset her.

I feel like screaming. I saw Georgina's mother at school one day when I went to pick Katy up. I felt like yelling at her. It's so rotten, so unfair! I kept thinking, Why, why, why should this have happened? What did Katy do to deserve it?—but what's the point? I know she is aware of her handicaps and it must be ghastly for her. We try to help her and do as much as we can but sometimes I must admit my patience wears thin. I don't get angry at her but it's oh so debilitating. Somehow this part is harder than the earlier months when practically every day we saw a little bit more improvement.

I've started praying again. Tessa told Ron that we must not stop our prayers and beliefs. Could it be that—oh horrible thought—there is some more serious damage that is only beginning to show itself now? I can't bear the idea. I am inured to pain. I feel as though a steel block has been erected around my feelings. I drink a lot of wine to blot out the pain. It is as if my soul has been anaesthetized. I want her back as she was. I know it's illogical to expect so much now, I know she *will* come back, but I can't bear the waiting. I want to help her more. *I want her back NOW!*

Three days later: Today Katy made a big breakthrough in terms of her activity. Although she complained of a sore throat and so didn't go to school, she was jumping about the house laughing—very energetic—crawling and climbing all over the sofas and drawing some very good pictures. It was a real joy to see her today. Dr Balfour-Lynn came to see her and according to Fiona was "amazed" by her latest progress. Perhaps Lillian Grant's strong nutritional programme, which she has been on for the past ten days and which is supposed to feed and nourish her new cells, is working. Or maybe it's just that she spent the weekend in the country with Ron and me, and even though she had behavioural problems she really loves the cosy country life. I realize how good it is for her too but it's not possible to live there all the time. Anyway, fingers crossed—Keep it up Katy!

THE TENTH MONTH

It's forty-three weeks since Katy's accident. I suppose it's something we have now adjusted to completely. It seems as though she has always been like this. "This", however, is a wonderful, sweet adorable child, who, if one had not known her before the accident, one would not realize was in any way different from any other child. She is, of course, still faintly clumsy in her movement, but her speech is as loud as before although somewhat slower. She controls her left hand quite expertly while writing but you can notice the slight shakiness if you look for it. After the first week of term her headmistress said how much confidence she has now. It is incredible for me to watch her lying on the floor on Saturday morning, watching

Tiswas, in her pink dressing-gown with her hair medium long and much blonder from the sun. She is leaning on her chin with her sturdy little legs crossed *exactly* as she looked forty-three weeks ago when I told her we were going to Paris.

The past couple of months have shown very slow but steady improvement. She works very hard at acrostics—those funny word-finding games. I find them impossible to do, but she can be enthralled by them for hours. She averages sixteen out of twenty in her spelling and dictation tests at school; before she was in the top two or three in her class and now she is in the middle section. I worry most about her short-term memory. Unless something has been written down by her teacher she can't remember it, and she gets terribly frustrated doing homework and sometimes Fiona has to help her with all of it. Richard Todd, with whom I am now doing a play, *Murder in Mind*, at Guildford, said that he was concussed for three days in the Army during the war and that his memory was bad for over a year. I'm sure Katy's will get better eventually—the question is, *when*?

Various events this month have alternately thrilled me to bits and depressed the hell out of me. The most thrilling thing was three weeks ago: I was playing a record and doing exercises in my bedroom when suddenly Katy, who had been watching me, started to do some incredibly graceful and dexterous ballet-cum-modern-jazz-cum-disco dancing. For nearly an hour she danced. Steps and movements that I couldn't believe she could do were executed with agility and precision, and with no trace of trembling or hesitation. She was fluid, expressive and magical. She watched herself in the full-length mirror in our bedroom and was obviously pleased with herself. I started to cry. It was almost as wonderful as when she first opened her eyes. She went upstairs to put on her ballet shoes and started *jetés*, and even tried to get *en pointe*. What was also amazing was that the dancing was totally synchronized to the different beats on the record. There was fast jazz, sensual slow Latin-American sounds, and rock-and-roll, and she was completely in time, moving as though she'd been rehearsing for weeks. I called Ron, who was in Los Angeles, and told him, and he was thrilled. But the strange thing is that although this happened nearly a month ago, and in spite of my asking, cajoling and pleading, she has *refused* to dance again. Why, I wonder. Ron says that the fact that she was able to do it once is a breakthrough and even if she doesn't do it for months, she has proved that she can.

THE ELEVENTH MONTH

Mr Illingworth came to see Katy. He hadn't seen her for three months and *again* was extremely surprised that she had improved so much. She was bored by being examined by him and couldn't wait to get away while he was asking her to do her "tricks"—she wanted to go and do her homework. Fortunately he said this was an excellent sign! He told me that with her type of brain injury the major part of the improvement occurs in the first six months after the accident. That is why he said in January, when I was so frightened by her idiosyncrasies, "What she is left with is what she is left with." He said he realized he had been wrong then, and he couldn't be happier that he *was* wrong. He thought it appeared she will get back to 98 or 99 per cent but maybe not a hundred per cent. This made me a tiny bit sad, but I suppose I shouldn't be greedy as we have got so much of her back. Without being cocky, Ron and I think she is the best child in the world!

I have been receiving three or four letters a week from desperate parents and friends of children and young adults now in comas. They ask for any advice and help I can give, and I try to do as much as I can. I know that a lot of the reasons why Katy has done so well are because of the constant stimulation,

144

care, love and patience Ron and I expended on her. That is why I want to try and help other parents who will be in this awful situation. I would like something lasting and valuable to come out of our terrible experiences, and that is why I've decided to publish this diary.

Katy was nine years old on 20th June. She had a "punk rock" party, which she had always wanted, but her hair is almost shoulder length now. I pulled bits of it up in bunches and tied them with black ribbons, and she wore a black leotard, a black mini-skirt and a pair of my black stockings. She whispered to me, "Black is a sexy colour." Milica and a friend from school, Helena, stayed with us the night before the party and I made them all up and took photographs. Katy looked sensational—Ron was completely knocked out by her. She is so beautiful.

About sixteen kids came to the party in the garden at our house in the country. We played grandmother's footsteps, musical bumps and musical statues. There was no trace of shyness or shakiness in Katy that day, but she became quite upset if she didn't win or was told she was out of one of the games. This was rather unnerving as she exhibited real prima-donna temper-tantrums. She did this several times when she didn't get her own way. After each outburst she apologized with enormous charm to her friends—all of whom, I'm relieved to see, like her a lot, even when she's being cranky. Kids are very understanding. All in all it was a good day. I remembered that on previous birthdays she had often gone over the top and behaved badly. But then many children do. Too much excitement, perhaps.

The great event of this month is that her tear ducts are working again. After ten months! Little tears coursed down her cheeks, and I was really happy even though she was crying. I made her taste her tears to see how salty they were, and then she laughed!

145

THE TWELFTH MONTH

I took Katy to see one of the best speech therapists specializing in brain-injured children in England. She had been recommended to us by Mr Illingworth. She gave Katy various tests—interesting and fun things mostly. She said her tongue was still not co-operating properly and she needed to do exercises for it. She also needed exercises for her immediate memory as she can't remember what she has just learned or heard. This, of course, is rather serious and is not something that is going to be cured overnight.

Katy's school Sports Day was held in Hyde Park on 2nd July. It was a day both Ron and I were dreading because in the past two years she had done so well. Last year she even won the sack race! I was a nervous wreck waiting for the first event in which Katy participated, which was, believe it or not, the egg-and-spoon race. I was amazed they could put her in it, as her two main physical problems are co-ordination and balance—and the "egg" was a ping-pong ball! Well, she really really tried. My heart went out to her, but of course the "egg" kept dropping and the children were only allowed to use the hand holding the spoon to pick it up. It fell lots of times (it was windy too) but she was absolutely determined to finish and gamely picked it up and went on again and again and again. She came last by a long way—all the other kids were back in their places by the time she had reached the finishing line. But she was so sweet and didn't seem too upset, just a little disappointed. Then she went in for the eighty-metre dash, in which I thought she was brilliant and very co-ordinated. Her running movements were excellent but since she has only been doing sports again at school since April, she was not as fast as the others and came third from last. This seemed to upset her enormously. I saw that she was with her little group in the centre of the field getting agitated. We tried to comfort her and take her to have an ice cream but she was in a really bad, angry, unhappy mood and refused to be comforted.

"This is the worst day and the worst year of my life!" she yelled, little face all red and cross. She is so competitive and loves to win, so her feelings of frustration were quite understandable. To make up for it, and to try and make her feel a bit better, I decided to go in for the mothers' eighty-metres and I came second! Katy was very pleased, and I realized how fit I must be, even after the strain of this year.

Then, to my horror, I saw that Katy was competing in the chariot race. This is where two kids, one's right leg tied to the other's left leg, carry two more kids on their backs. Ten of these little groups were competing. My heart was in my mouth because Katy couldn't possibly be co-ordinated or strong enough to do this, particularly since she had her left leg tied. Naturally she fell down and they all fell on top of her and she bent her leg back and cried bitter tears. I was disturbed that the school had let her enter for this, but perhaps they thought that competing with others would be better for her than just standing on the sidelines feeling left out. It is important that her school-mates treat her as absolutely normal.

After the Sports Day she was in a very bad mood for several days and even went back to walking stiffly again. She wants so much to do well and even when we encourage her, if she doesn't do well at something it's a step backwards in her mind. On the plus side she has started playing the piano. She came back from a weekend in Edinburgh with Fiona, who said she was really good and very musical. We bought her a piano for her birthday present which we keep at the country house and she plays it constantly. From the first tune which we heard sixty times a day, she has now progressed to knowing three—so things are looking up.

We have rented South Street to Michael and Shakira Caine

for two months as we are planning on spending the summer in the country house. Katy is quite happy going to school on the Dorking train in the morning, although she gets very nervous if she thinks she's going to be late. She is so fastidious and everything must be just so, but then she was always like that. It's the last bit of recovery which seems to be taking so long. We *think* there is improvement, and of course there is—all the time—but then we are hit by the realization that there is still a way to go. How long will it be now, I wonder? I can't predict any more.

She loves the country and the sunshine. We will take her for a sunny holiday in Marbella soon. Dr Eppel still feels also that we should spend the winter in California if we can.

My hopes of Katy being one hundred per cent by the 2nd August deadline we set for her are obviously not going to come true. Soon it will be a year since the accident. In some ways time has gone incredibly fast. Looking at her sometimes I simply cannot believe that this dreadful event could possibly have happened to her. Within the last couple of weeks since the school holidays began, there have been hours at a time when it hasn't even crossed my mind that she is any different. However, there are other times when I see her disabilities clearly, especially her shakiness which happens particularly when she's tired. My heart bleeds for her. She is so intelligent she must wonder why, why, why does my left hand shake when I want to control it? She has become the dearest, most loving child in the world. When Ron and I were having a minor argument the other day she grabbed our hands and said, "Promise me that you'll never *ever* get divorced!"

Her end-of-term report was *excellent*—so good that I took her headmistress out to lunch to find out if they had made some of it up!

148

NAME: Katyana Kass
FORM: IV
AGE: 9.1
Summer Term, 1981
Attendance: Fair, absent ten days. Punctuality: Very good

ENGLISH
Spelling—Katy's everyday spelling is good and she works hard for her weekly tests. She is extremely articulate, both orally and in her written work. Her grammar is good and comprehension shows intelligence. Sentence construction and content show thought and originality.
Essay—Imagination is very good and she usually writes at length, sometimes without regard for punctuation or paragraphing and breaks all the rules. Nevertheless, when all this is rectified she should do quite well.
Reading—Katy has made excellent progress in her reading but she needs to speak up more.

MATHEMATICS
Tables—fairly good. Katy's ability to retain mathematical concepts has improved enormously during the term and she is regaining her former high standards of accuracy. Her work is always well presented.

HISTORY
Katy has progressed well this term, she is a diligent worker and produces clear, neat and factual essays. Illustrations are pertinent and well drawn.

GEOGRAPHY
Katy tries hard and has had some success in atlas work this term. Her maps and diagrams are neat and clear.

149

LANGUAGE:
French: Good, Katyana shows potential, she is beginning to grasp the principles and can apply them intelligently.

SCIENCE
Katy has tried very hard to keep detailed written notes and her drawings are neat and accurate. She enjoys practical work.

ART
Katy shows potential in drawing and picture composition.

MUSIC
Katy shows care and sensitivity in all she does. She takes an enthusiastic part in class and enjoys singing and instrumental work.

GAMES
Katy enjoys sport and participates enthusiastically in all games. Her co-ordination has improved enormously but it is still a little slow.

GENERAL REPORT
A pleasing term. Katy has worked hard and produced work of a high standard. Her memory has improved considerably. She is a helpful, enthusiastic and popular member of the class who involves herself well in all activities. She has a mature attitude to her work. Presentation is excellent. Judging by her present standard of achievement it should not be long before she catches up with the children of her own age-group.

Her headmistress assured me that everything that she and the staff at school had written was completely true. "Although," she said with a twinkle, "we did do several drafts, as we know that the children always look at their reports and we wanted to be spot on and encourage Katyana."

I quote the report as I think it is extremely impressive and shows Katy's determination, absolute will-power and desire to improve. I was concerned that she may not be able to keep up next term, and that—oh horrors—we may have to put her in a special school, as the speech therapist says that her memory and learning capacity need a lot of work. The head-mistress *assured* me wholeheartedly that this was nonsense and that her learning capacity was such that she had no doubt *whatsoever* that not only could Katy keep up with the work, but that she would be able to pass the exam to enter the secondary school in two years when she would be eleven. She was most impressed by Katy's overall efforts, although she did say that she goes off into a sort of daze sometimes, as though she were completely disorientated, but she soon snaps out of it and gets back to herself again. She said how much the staff and teachers cared for Katy and, without wanting to make her feel different, they were still aware of her problems. Katy gets round many of these problems herself. When it was her turn to clear the tables, for example, which they do in alphabetical order, instead of taking nine or ten plates together which the other kids do, she cleverly took only three or four at a time. Smart cookie! She has also started keeping a scrapbook of the forthcoming Royal Wedding. She admires Lady Diana.

ONE YEAR

Marbella
The one-year anniversary of Katy's accident has now passed. No, she is not a hundred per cent recovered *yet*, and this has caused Ron and me many bitter, anguished hours. However as I look at her now in her chic khaki shorts, navy blue T-shirt with a Snoopy on it, lying on a sun bed, reading *One Hundred and One Dalmatians*, chewing gum, with her long tanned legs and her long blonde streaked hair, my heart overflows with joy.

We are so lucky, Ron and I. She came back from the brink of death to a full existence. From the time we knew she would live (although as *what* we couldn't ever really bear to contemplate) we worked our asses off against all the odds to make her a whole child again. I realize, on looking back over the past year, that Ron and I gave each other the courage and moral support to carry on. Without him I couldn't have done it. His strength gave me mine. We had a blind, all-consuming faith and belief that she would be ours again—as she was: our Katy, funny, beautiful, vital, clever. She is almost there now. At dinner the other night she started to do imitations of various school-friends of hers, mimicking their accents and their mannerisms, and she had Ron, Fiona and me in stitches. She is quite a clever mimic, mocking the American drawl of Ron's mother, and the cockney whine of some kids at school. There are still many problems to overcome. She is shy and reticent with strangers. She drags her left foot slightly when she walks. Her speech is a little monotonous and slow but her voice projection has returned. Her right pupil is still two-thirds dilated. Her left hand is still shaky. She has a touch of forgetfulness. But all of this is unimportant. It is only one year, after all. It may take one or two years more. We don't care. We know it will happen for her eventually.

Joan Axelrod phoned me last week to tell me about her son Jonathan. At the age of fourteen he was kicked in the head on a football field in California and went into a coma for several weeks. The Axelrods were told there was no hope, that he would never be normal again. The doctors wanted to perform a frontal lobotomy but the Axelrods refused, as the chances of coming out of an operation like that were usually pretty dim in those days (about twenty years ago). The Axelrods spent two years doing with Jonathan what Ron and I did with Katy, but his progress was very slow and he had to go to special schools as he had problems with reading, writing etc., and also behavioural problems. Today Jonathan Axelrod is one of the heads of a television company in California. It just goes to show what the power of positivity can do. However long it takes, I know Katy is going to be fine. She is such a wonderful spirit. So kind, sweet, sensitive and loving.

Two weeks ago Simon Williams, Lucy Fleming, Ron and I were having a drink together after the Berkeley Square Ball when a woman came over and started chatting, asking all sorts of questions about Katy. I was answering them all very positively and happily, babbling on about how lucky we were, what a miracle Katy is and so on, and suddenly I became aware of Lucy next to me, and how she must be feeling, hearing my joy. Her daughter Flora drowned six months ago. *Nothing* can be harder to bear for a parent than the loss of their child. My heart went out to her and I almost felt guilty that God had spared Katy but taken Flora. Life is hard. Life is cruel. Life is not fair. Those words were spoken to me so many times in the hospital. Now I realize the truth in them. But I also realize that life is beautiful. Life is a wonderful and joyous gift which those of us who are lucky enough to have our health, and the health and support of those we love, should cherish and appreciate infinitely more than most of us do.

Ron and I got our Katy back. Some parents perhaps will not be so lucky, but many, I hope, will find some words of help and encouragement in what I have written and will be able to cope with the tragedy that you think can never happen to you.

Epilogue

LONDON: *Christmas Eve 1981*

"She has come a long, long way." Robin Illingworth spoke those words to us in the hospital fifteen months ago when Katy could barely sit up, let alone walk or talk. I thought then how far she *had* come. What, naturally, I wasn't aware of was the immensity of the road ahead of her. Ron and I were so lucky to have such a complete optimism and conviction about our daughter's recovery. I had a sort of child-like naïvety that somehow total recovery would happen overnight. Well, it didn't. I still haven't eaten any chocolate, even though Tara tried to make me have some today. "Look at Katy, Mummy. Look at that little girl. She's perfect! She's completely *better!*" Katy was twirling around on a stool chattering on the phone non-stop to Fiona in Scotland. She was wearing a new red sweater and had a beret over her long streaky blonde hair. We had just returned from California and her face was tanned. She looked exquisite.

Tara is right. She *is* perfect. She *is* better. Not yet completely —but she will be. She is enrolled in a special programme of physical education at the school she has been attending in California, where we are living while I work on the television series *Dynasty*. Living in California has done wonders for her. Last month we took her to Roger Whittaker's concert and he dedicated a song to her called "My Little Miracle"—that she most certainly is. Her goal is to be able to do a cartwheel by 30th March, which is Ron's birthday. She covers up her minor

155

disabilities well. They are only physical, thank God. Mentally she is perfect. She is learning the piano and can read music now, and does so excellently; she takes ballet (against her will) and is improving; she has started tennis lessons and is enthusiastic; her swimming is superb; her school-work is excellent, and her American teacher says she is a dream and she wishes she had more like her in class! She beats me at backgammon constantly, she writes poetry and draws beautifully, she plays word-games and gets everything right; she is as busy as a bee all day long, and watches television only for the particular programmes she admires. She sings like an angel. She performed several Christmas songs with her class at the end of term. She sang so well that I asked her to sing tonight after Christmas dinner for our guests. She was shy at first but her voice rang out pure and clear without hesitation. All of us at the table—Ron, Bill and Hazel, Tara and her boyfriend, and Rod and Maggie—were tremendously moved by this moment. With the red candles flickering behind her blonde head and the snow-filled vista of the garden, featuring the snowman that she and Tara had made, in the background, she was the most wonderful Christmas present we could ever hoped to have had.

ONWARD!